Robert C. Scaer, MD

The Body Bears the Burden
Trauma, Dissociation, and Disease

Pre-publication
REVIEWS,
COMMENTARIES,
EVALUATIONS . . .

"Therapists of various clinical disciplines are now becoming increasingly aware that traumatic disorders involve severe dysregulations of both mind and body. This means that advances in treatment must be based on very recent models that integrate the psychological and biological realms. In light of the current explosion of recent interdisciplinary findings across an array of scientific disciplines, this is a formidable task. Dr. Robert Scaer is in an extraordinary position to address this problem. In addition to possessing more clinical experience in treating traumatic disorders than any other currently practicing neurologist, he is also deeply steeped in a number of scientific literatures that are now producing knowledge directly relevant to a deeper understanding of the psychobiological manifestations of these disorders.

In this remarkable work, Dr. Scaer provides clinically relevant descriptions of the mind/body dysfunctions of both the central and autonomic nervous systems of traumatized patients. In addition, he offers current ideas about the critical role of early affect regulation and child abuse in the pathogenesis of traumatic disorders. Even more than a comprehensive overview, the author presents an integrated psychoneurobiological model of the underlying mechanisms of trauma pathology, which he demonstrates in numerous case histories and applies to various trauma therapies. This is a creative, cutting-edge work, the product of Dr. Scaer's rigorous scientific perspective and extraordinarily intuitive clinical skills. It is valuable as both a guidebook to the individual clinician, as well as a theoretical mapping on which to build more effective treatment models of the traumatic disorders of brain/mind/body."

Allan N. Schore, PhD
Assistant Clinical Professor,
Department of Psychiatry,
University of California
at Los Angeles
School of Medicine

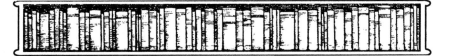

The Haworth Medical Press®
An Imprint of The Haworth Press, Inc.

The Body Bears the Burden
*Trauma, Dissociation,
and Disease*

THE HAWORTH MEDICAL PRESS
New, Recent, and Forthcoming Titles of Related Interest

The Body Bears the Burden
Trauma, Dissociation, and Disease

Robert C. Scaer, MD

The Haworth Medical Press®
An Imprint of The Haworth Press, Inc.
New York • London • Oxford

Published by

The Haworth Medical Press®, an imprint of The Haworth Press, Inc., 10 Alice Street, Binghamton, NY 13904-1580

Medicine is an ever-changing science. As new research and clinical experience broaden our knowledge, changes in treatment and drug therapy are required. While many suggestions for drug usages or treatment regimens are made herein, the book is intended for educational purposes only, and the author, editor, and publisher do not accept liability in the event of negative consequences incurred as a result of information presented in this book. We do not claim that this information is necessarily accurate by the rigid, scientific standard applied for medical proof, and therefore make no warranty, expressed or implied, with respect to the material herein contained. Therefore the patient is urged to check the product information sheet included in the package of each drug he or she plans to administer to be certain the protocol followed is not in conflict with the manufacturer's inserts. When a discrepancy arises between these inserts and information in this book, the physician is encouraged to use his or her best professional judgement.

Cover design by Marylouise E. Doyle.

Library of Congress Cataloging-in-Publication Data

Scaer, Robert C.
    The body bears the burden : trauma, dissociation, and disease / Robert C. Scaer.
        p.   cm.
    Includes bibliographical references and index.
    ISBN 0-7890-1245-6 (hard) — ISBN 0-7890-1246-4 (soft)
    1. Post-traumatic stress disorder—Treatment. 2. Bioenergetic psychotherapy. 3. Mind and body therapies. 4. Somatoform disorders—Treatment. I. Title.

RC552.P67 S2236 2000
616.85'21—dc21

00-047213

ABOUT THE AUTHOR

Robert C. Scaer, MD, earned a BA in psychology and an MD at the University of Rochester, NY. He served his internship and a residency in neurology at the University of Colorado School of Medicine. He served as Associate Clinical Professor of Neurology at the University of Colorado Health Sciences Center, Denver. In addition, he has spent more than thirty years practicing medicine.

For twenty years he was Medical Director of Rehabilitation Services at Boulder Memorial Hospital and the Mapleton Center in Boulder, Colorado. He also served as Medical Director of Pain Management Services at the Mapleton Center, a Division of Boulder Community Hospital.

Dr. Scaer is a Diplomate of the American Board of Psychiatry and Neurology and a certified member of the American Society of Neuro Rehabilitation. As well as being a member of many professional societies, he is a Fellow of the American Academy of Neurology. Dr. Scaer has served on accreditation committees for rehabilitation facilities and has a lengthy list of publications and presentations to his credit.

CONTENTS

Foreword

About a century ago, scientists became aware of the existence of memories that are different from the memories of everyday experience. Ordinarily, events are remembered as stories that change over time and that do not evoke intense emotions and sensations. However, since time immemorial there have been records of people being tormented by memories that fill them with feelings of irreparable loss, and sensations of fright and horror. The neurologists and psychiatrists at the end of the nineteenth century elucidated the nature of posttraumatic conditions and showed that elements of the past were relived with an immediate sensory and emotional intensity that makes victims feel as if it were occurring all over again. While trauma-related emotions and sensations endured, however, conscious knowledge of the event itself was sometimes absent. They discovered that, paradoxically, even though vivid elements of the trauma intrude insistently in the form of flashbacks and nightmares, many traumatized people have a great deal of difficulty relating precisely what has happened. They often experience sensory elements of the trauma without being able to make sense out of what they are feeling or seeing. These mysterious combinations of remembering emotions and sensations, while forgetting the origin and the content, were called "repression" and "dissociation."

These early scientists hypothesized that these amnesias and intrusive re-experiences were the result of severely paralyzing fears in response to terrifying life events. For example, the "father of neurology," Jean Martin Charcot, noted that: "The patient . . . does not preserve any recollection, or he preserves it in a vague manner. . . . Questions addressed to him upon this point are attended with no result. He knows nothing or almost nothing." These early students of the effects of fear-related trauma noted that the loss of memory is not merely an inability to recall the specific event, but, more relevant, a lack of capacity for sustained thought, and for continued application to work. These patients had problems with attention, and were easily fatigued.

xi

They also noted that traumatic memories are intricately connected with one's sense of "self" and "self-awareness," and that, when the fear, fright, and hyperarousal that accompany trauma interfere with forming a well-defined, verbal memory of events, people lose their sense of themselves, start feeling helpless and look to others for reassurance.

At the beginning of the last century, the great physiologist Walter Cannon proposed that traumatic emotions constitute phases of physiological mobilization in an internal environment that is perpetually striving to adjust itself, through the actions of the sympathetic nervous system and the endocrines, to changes and challenges in the organism's external environment: "[T]he bodily changes which occur in the intense emotional states—such as fear and fury occur as results of sympathetic discharges, and are in the highest degree serviceable to the organism in the struggle for existence. Thus are the body's reserves—the stored adrenalin, and the accumulated sugar—called forth for instant service; thus is the blood shifted to nerves and muscles that may have to bear the brunt of struggle; thus is the heart set rapidly beating to speed the circulation; and thus also, are the activities of the digestive organs for the time abolished (Cannon 1914: 275). Cannon pointed out how sometimes what starts out as a survival mechanism (mobilization) is transformed into its opposite to such a degree that it may even lead to "'Voodoo' Death."

When people develop PTSD, the replaying of the trauma leads to sensitization: with every replay of the trauma there is an increasing level of distress. In those individuals, the traumatic event, which started out as a social and interpersonal process, develops secondary biological consequences that are hard to reverse once they become entrenched. Because these patients have intolerable sensations and feelings, their tendency is to actively avoid them. Mentally, they split off or "dissociate" these feelings; physically, their bodies tighten and brace against them. They seem to live under the assumption that if they feel those sensations and feelings, they will overwhelm them forever. These are patients who rely on medications, drugs, and alcohol to make these sensations and feelings go away, because they have lost confidence that they can learn to tolerate them without outside help. The fear of being consumed by these "terrible" feelings leads them to believe that only not feeling them will make them go away.

Allan Young has pointed out that implicit traumatic memories, avoidance, and helplessness challenge two core foundations of the Western consciousness: free will and self-determination. The emotional dependency of traumatized people, and their inability to utilize the help offered, in turn, evoke frustration, contempt, and even sadism in those to whom the victims turn for help.

Most whiplash victims have emotional symptoms: they may feel numb or detached, while experiencing anxiety related to automobile travel. This may progress to actual panic attacks when other cars drive too closely, approach rapidly behind them, or when they drive by the scene of their accident. Many suffer from flashbacks of the accident. Many also suffer from exaggerated startle responses to loud noises. Bright lights and loud or unpleasant noises may become intolerable, and cause anxiety and "overload." They may wake up in the middle of the night with severe anxiety, sometimes accompanied by memories of nightmares. If enough of these symptoms appear, they may receive the diagnosis of post-traumatic stress disorder (PTSD), although most of them suffer from only a few of these symptoms.

Traditionally, the symptoms of traumatic brain injury have been ascribed to injury to the brain and the tissues of the head. Post-concussion syndrome, however, tends to follow minor brain injury much more often than more severe brain injury. Ironically, the long-term disability after six to twelve months post-accident is greater in mild concussion than in moderate brain injury in which the patient does not remember the accident. The mechanisms of minor traumatic brain injury are generally thought to be due to the tearing or stretching of axons (axonal shearing) due to forces related to excessive changes in velocity of the head during the acceleration/deceleration of the head during the movement of whiplash. However, studies have shown, on the one hand, that actual head impact is not necessary to cause axonal shearing and, on the other, that there is a remarkable consistency in the cognitive symptoms of the traumatized patients, regardless of the specific impact.

As with other traumatized patients described over the past 120 years, traumatic brain injury patients suffer from a reduced rate of information processing, increased reaction time, and problems with divided attention. They are distracted, and have problems with concentration. They will forget events, appointments, and things they have said to other people. One of the most persistent and debilitating symptoms is pervasive fatigue: they "shut down." All of these symptoms are compatible with the abnormalities found in neuroimaging studies of traumatized patients.

In this book, Scaer proposes to discard the concept of physical and structural injuries to the spine, jaw, and brain as the model for whiplash-based injury, and instead proposes that the whiplash experience is a model of traumatization, with long-standing and at times permanent neurophysiological and neurochemical changes in the brain that are experience-based, rather than injury-based. Scaer proposes that these changes are triggered by a cascade of neural impulses and neurotransmitters precipitated by a continuous state of intense arousal alternating with recurrence of the freeze response resulting in turn from an unresolved perceived life threat in a state of relative helplessness. The depth of memory is a function of the arousal or emotional content of the experience that accompanied the event. The brain readily forms procedural memories of intense emotional events. These are acquired and stored without the necessary involvement of conscious memory centers serving declarative memory, such as the hippocampus and prefrontal cortex.

The basic premise is that whiplash injury is a traumatic experience that represents a threat to the very survival of the individual. In this definition, the meaning of the event may be as important to the traumatized person as what actually physically happens to that person. This is a dramatic departure from the long-standing and traditional concept of whiplash as spinal injury. It presents, however, a compelling and logical theory, bringing together the diverse elements of the whiplash syndrome into a cohesive whole.

To understand and properly treat these symptoms clinicians need to appreciate what happens to a body frozen in fear. Post-concussion syndromes need to be understood as representing disassociated imprints of traumatic experience—physical sensations, panic, and helplessness—that have overwhelmed these patients. Fighting against and/or hiding from unpleasant or painful sensations and feelings will generally make things worse. The more feelings need to be avoided, the more energy is spent on keeping them at bay—energy that should have been used for feeling alive and open to new experiences. What is not felt remains unchanged or gains in inward pressure, which forces people to step up their methods of avoidance. This is the sort of vicious cycle that trauma creates. Abandoned feelings call out for attention from the growing shadow of existence. Treatment must aim at putting these disjointed sensations together. Doing this involves coaxing them gently to begin to feel and tolerate the sensations that once overwhelmed them.

Bessel A. van der Kolk, MD
Medical Director, the Trauma Center
Professor of Psychiatry
Boston University School of Medicine

Preface

When Beth first came to my office, she brought her best friend, a nurse, "to interpret for her." Beth was quite guarded, almost suspicious, with wide, frightened eyes. She sat with her arms held tightly at her side, holding a handkerchief, her head forward, and her shoulders raised and tense. Her forehead was furrowed, and at twenty-five, she looked closer to forty. She said that she had suffered whiplash in an accident, and was not getting any better. A friend had referred her to me because of my interest in motor vehicle accident-related injuries. Her insurance company was beginning to question her treatment, since the accident had occurred at speeds of 5 to 10 mph. No damage occurred to either car, and the driver of the other car suffered no injuries. Beth, on the other hand, continued to suffer from terrible neck and shoulder pain, numbness of her right arm, disabling headaches, and temporomandibular joint syndrome. Six months of chiropractic treatment and massage therapy brought her only temporary relief from pain, and a dental splint only slightly helped her morning headaches. Recently she developed severe pain in her right hip and buttock, with the pain radiating down the back of her leg. X rays and MRIs failed to show any cause for her spinal or leg pain.

Since the accident, Beth had also experienced worsening problems of distraction and an inability to concentrate. Her memory was terrible, and she would constantly go somewhere and forget what she had intended to do. She had recently started to drive again, and would travel to some familiar place in town, and on arriving, realize that she could not remember how she got there. She would stumble over words, say the wrong word for what she meant, and then feel stupid. She even had developed a strange stutter whenever she was stressed. She constantly made errors in her checkbook.

Worst of all, since the accident, she had become panicky when traveling in a car, especially as a passenger. Her heart would pound for no reason. She had become edgy and irritable, and jumped at every loud sound. Thoughts and images of the accident kept popping into her mind, producing distraction and anxiety. Although she finally was able to fall asleep without drugs, she kept waking fully aroused, sometimes with a racing heart, sometimes with dreams of the accident or of being threatened with no means of escape. During the day, she was exhausted by every physical and mental effort, and had dropped out of her master's program in clinical social work. Her extreme sensitivity to almost any stimulus had resulted in her isolation from almost all of her prior social activities.

She admitted that at times she was worried that she might have a brain tumor. She experienced dizziness when she moved her head too quickly, kept losing her balance and bumping into things, and noticed that her vision blurred whenever she moved her focus from one object to another. Reading caused blurring of vision and a headache. Only an MRI of her head reassured her that she had no diseases of her brain.

As I do with all of my motor vehicle accident (MVA) patients, I asked her in detail about past traumatic life experiences. Similar to many of my patients, she was very open and candid and willing to share with me what must have been a hellish nightmare of her childhood. She was supported in this discussion by the confidante and friend who had accompanied her. From the age of six through twelve, she was visited twice each week after bedtime by her brother, who was older by seven years. As if by ritual, he would painfully twist her right arm behind her back as she lay in bed on her stomach, pull down her panties, and rape her. Any sound by her would result in his beating her, or covering her head with a pillow as he abused her. She never told her parents for fear of punishment by her verbally abusive alcoholic father. At age nineteen, her brother ran away from home and the abuse stopped. During college, memories and panic related to the abuse resurfaced, and she underwent years of counseling, which enabled her to "put it all behind her." She obtained her degree, and, prior to the accident, had been pursuing a graduate degree with the goal of becoming a social worker.

When I examined Beth, she was quite guarded and defensive, exhibiting what one might call "exaggerated pain behavior." She manifested "give-away" weakness of her right arm and leg, and "stocking and glove" anesthesia of these extremities, as well as loss of sensation to pin prick over the entire right side of her head and face. Remarkably, however, her right hand was slightly cooler to touch than the left, and patterns of hair growth revealed subtle but definite thinning over the right side of her scalp. Her neck was quite resistant to passive movement, and neck extension immediately caused her to become nauseated. Tightness, tenderness, and trigger points were prominent in her neck, jaw, and shoulder girdle muscles, and straight leg raising caused pain in her right hip and tingling of her right foot.

The story of Beth's whiplash experience is a compilation of symptoms seen consistently in thousands of my patients who have suffered injuries in MVAs. These unusual and multisystemic symptoms are so universal and consistent from patient to patient that they either constitute a vast medicolegal conspiracy to defraud the auto insurance industry, or a remarkably consistent and reproducible clinical syndrome. The whiplash syndrome has been a source of controversy, confusion, derision, and misunderstanding for most of its described existence. There is no question that it is indeed a syndrome, defined as "The aggregate of signs and symptoms associated with any morbid process, and constituting together the picture of the disease."[1]

The "picture of the disease" in this case is a diverse constellation of symptoms consisting of pain, neurologic symptoms, cognitive impairment, and emotional complaints. Each specific symptom and group of symptoms is remarkably similar from person to person, suggesting a unique and common cause. The defense bar and a substantial number of physicians would assert that this remarkable similarity is related to the phenomenon of secondary gain, and the sophisticated coaching of the plaintiff bar. Doubt is cast upon this assertion by the fact that few of these patients seem to recover after settlement of their case, even for substantial sums of money. The "green poultice" is more myth than reality.

A real dilemma in assessing the cause and validity of this syndrome, however, is the fact that it frequently occurs in a setting of an insufficient velocity and force of collision to logically cause bodily injury. Another major dilemma is the diffuse and diverse nature of the symptoms. The whiplash syndrome seems to affect a great portion of the victim's conscious existence. It impairs the mind (cognitive and attention deficits), the body (severe and widespread pain, vertigo, visual impairment, paresthesia), and the spirit (anxiety, insomnia, depression). One of the most poignant complaints I hear is that the patient has "lost who I once was." And years later, although blessedly much healing has taken place, most patients feel permanently and irrevocably changed by their experience. No amount of financial reward cures them of their recurrent episodes of unexplained pain or their altered sense of self. Even relatively minor life conflicts and stresses seem to throw them back into the distraction and confusion, the jitteriness and arousal, and the familiar tightening and spasm of the same groups of neck and shoulder muscles they know so well.

For years I have struggled with the inconsistencies between the physical injuries and the resulting diffuse and disabling symptoms experienced by patients after MVAs. I have searched the scientific literature on whiplash, much of which seeks to explain from a biomechanical standpoint the injuries to ligaments, discs, muscles, nerves, and brain cells and fibers. In courtroom testimony, I have struggled to justify the fact that an individual could have suffered permanent injuries to the brain and spine from a 10 mph rear-end collision, in the face of contrary testimony by accident-reconstruction engineers and the powerful weight of common sense. How could one person, knocked unconscious for an hour in a football game, be left with only minimal cognitive impairment three years later, while another, rear-ended at 10 mph, with damage only to the bumper, be effectively cognitively disabled three years later? Why are professional racecar drivers not disabled early in their careers from whiplash?

The first clue, I believe, lies in the *meaning* of the event during which the injury occurred. One tends not to develop the diverse and disabling symptoms described previously unless the injury occurs in a state of relative helplessness. A second clue lies in the life history of specific traumatic events, especially those experienced in childhood. I have found that the severity of a person's whiplash-related symptoms strongly correlates with his or her cumulative load of traumatic life experiences before the accident occurred. These experiences may be incredibly varied. They will be discussed in more detail in Chapter 9.

Another clue lies in the fact that all of the symptoms commonly seen in the whiplash syndrome may occur with remarkable similarity in other severely traumatic events not associated with physical injury. Examples include natural disasters, exposure to warfare, and social trauma (assault, kidnapping, rape). Symptoms following these traumatic events are generally attributed to post-traumatic stress disorder (PTSD), a purely psychiatric diagnosis. Much of the medical literature tends to ignore that often dramatic physical symptoms, including bowel disorders, myofascial pain, and cognitive impairment, accompany PTSD in a fashion often identical to that experienced in the whiplash syndrome. We therefore seem to be dealing with a syndrome affecting all aspects of a person's being, including body, mind, and spirit. This posttraumatic syndrome is produced by threat, shock, or injury that occurs in a state of helplessness, and the neurophysiological changes triggered by these experiences are somehow stored in a person's unconscious memory in a cumulative manner along with other such life experiences. Accumulation of traumatic life experiences then leads to a condition of increasing vulnerability and decreased resiliency to further trauma.

The somatic and emotional consequences of traumatic stress are generally misunderstood by members of the mainstream medical profession, who refer to the resulting constellation of symptoms as psychosomatic or psychological. And yet, it is clear that this syndrome is common and is probably represented in all societies. It may well account for many of the unexplained and poorly managed chronic illnesses that afflict us, and perhaps constitute the major source of visits to the physician's office.

The journey that led to this book began when Marcus Kurek, one of the physical therapists in the chronic pain treatment program that I direct, referred me to the writings of Peter Levine, psychologist and traumatologist. Levine developed his model of treatment of traumatized individuals from his observations of animals in the wild, noting that prey animals, although repeatedly threatened, did not seem to develop behaviors similar to traumatized human beings. He noted that when prey animals are no longer able to flee or fight, they enter the freeze, or immobility, response. During this peculiar period of suspended animation, all of the neurochemical events associated with the fight/flight response persist, including a high state of activation of the limbic system, and both sympathetic and parasympathetic limbs of the autonomic nervous system. If the prey animal survives, it will arouse, and then seem to discharge the fight/flight energy through trembling, perspiring, and deeply breathing, effectively "completing" the truncated somatic and autonomic activities associated with flight. Levine noted that humans, although frequently freezing in the face of threat, seldom go through this discharge of retained fight/flight energy, perhaps because of their highly developed cognitive brain centers that tend to suppress much instinctual behavior, or because of acquired patterns of acculturation. Abnormal storage of this intense state of arousal in selected brain centers then leads to the syndrome of traumatization that he describes in his writings.[2]

I realized at the time that behavior and sensations of the freeze response typified the immediate postaccident experience of my whiplash patients—a state of shock, numbing, immobility, and even depersonalization. Persistence of this response explained the remarkable delay in the onset of pain, cognitive impairment, and emotional symptoms seen in many of my patients. It also explained why many of my patients began to deteriorate weeks and even months after the accident. Finally, it explained why symptoms did not improve and disappear, but rather kept returning after hundreds of therapy treatments; why imaging studies seldom explained the cause of spinal soft tissue pain; and why so few of my patients recovered after their litigation was settled.

Since that moment of enlightenment, I have seen hundreds of victims of MVAs in a new light, taken detailed trauma histories, and begun to prescribe treatment programs emphasizing trauma therapy whenever possible. I have taken my ideas to the major auto insurance companies to enlist support in this area of treatment and in research; and received a predictably negative reception. In this process, I also began to examine and study victims of trauma with a new perspective, and started to correlate physical symptoms and syndromes with the burgeoning literature on the physiology of PTSD. Viewed in this context, I recognized subtle but consistent physical changes in my patients who have been labeled with the diagnosis of somatization, conversion, and secondary gain. The consistency of these findings among patients and their startling correlation with concepts of altered autonomic physiology has led me to the inescapable conclusion that clinical syndromes previously categorized as "nonphysiological," "psychosomatic," or "functional" may be based on demonstrable dynamic neurophysiological changes in the brain. These in turn may cause subtle but observable changes in the symptomatic body region. I now realize that the concept of whiplash remains only one small example of the pervasive physical, mental, and emotional devastation of traumatic stress.

I realize that I am treading on the dangerously thin divide separating the slippery slopes of the brain and the mind—time will undoubtedly prove that I have slipped a few times. As a neurologist, pursuing the topic of a psychiatric illness has presented a dilemma and a challenge. In presenting my evolving theories to my medical colleagues, I have predictably been met with skepticism that a dramatic physical syndrome with numerous, apparently disparate features could have its roots solely in a supposedly psychological event. Colleagues in the behavioral fields have been more receptive, but have still struggled with my contention that peripheral physical symptoms of conversion hysteria have a distinct physiological substrate, and are not solely manifestations of psychological dynamics.

Despite the medical community giving increasing lip service to rejecting Cartesian dualism, current psychosomaticists and holistic physicians continue to view "exaggerated" affective states and "nonphysiological" physical symptoms and findings as derived from psychological causes. Descartes, in fact, was probably not the author of our current concept of mind/body dualism.[3] In his treatise, *Meditation IV,* "Of the Existence of Material Things, and of the Real Distinction Between the Soul and the Body of Man," he argues that the soul in relationship to the body is "very closely united to it, and so to speak so intermingled with it that . . . [they] seem to compose . . . one whole."[4] In addition, in *The Passions of the Soul,* Descartes attributes a series of states of the mind to physical alterations of the body preceding or accompanying these mental states.[5] However, in *Passions,* Descartes indeed proposes that anger, joy, and other intense emotional states may be a *consequence* of somatic or material physical states, but not a cause of them[5] (p. 326). This specific theoretical departure from his contemporary colleagues may well have destined Descartes to be the scapegoat for the evolution of the concept of separation of mind and body in contemporary medicine.

As a result, Descartes has been blamed for a concept and language placing emotional and unexplainable somatic complaints in the intangible category of *psychological* events, and those symptoms and signs that we can measure by our tangible physiological images and measures in the category of *physiological* diseases.

Although we have come to accept that prolonged emotional distress appears to have adverse health effects on the body, our rigid application of the scientific method to the relatively primitive science of medicine has tended to blind us to the subtleties of somatic manifestations of emotional states. In the absence of sophisticated imaging studies and laboratory measures, the early pioneers of medical science relied on keen senses of observation, and the necessity of deriving their diagnoses from the history and physical examination alone. They derived their insights and wisdom from case studies and experience, and the cumulative knowledge taught to them by their patients. Many of the insights presented in this book also derive from clinical observations that patients alone can provide, built on a base of knowledge gleaned from the psychophysiological literature on traumatic stress. The result is not an affirmation of the mind/body connection, but of the mind/brain/body continuum.

Finally, through this journey, my belief that patient education is a powerful therapeutic tool has been greatly enhanced. Altering the threat of the unknown by informing and educating the patient changes the body's stress response and promotes healing. Many whiplash victims suffer almost as much from the dismissal and invalidation by the medical and insurance industries as they do from the effects of the accident itself. Providing them with a rational and comprehensive explanation for their symptoms is strong medicine. The obvious enlightenment experienced by my patients, the gratitude expressed, and the improved response to therapy resulting from detailed education, have all inspired and strengthened me in writing this book. Although this is not a book likely to be easily understood by the lay public, I have attempted to gear it to general professionals in the fields of rehabilitation and psychotherapy, patient care, and general medical practice. I hope that it will prove to be valuable to their understanding of this challenging group of patients.

Acknowledgments

In 1996 I came across the writings of psychologist and traumatologist Peter Levine. I recognized in his description of the phenomenon of the freeze response in animals many of the symptoms and features of my whiplash victims immediately after an accident. The persisting symptoms in my patients who failed to recover after prolonged treatment matched in remarkable detail the late effects of trauma described by Levine. I would specifically refer the reader to his recent book, *Waking the Tiger: Healing Trauma,* North Atlantic Press, 1997, for a detailed discussion of Dr. Levine's theories and treatment method for trauma. These ideas led me to redefine symptoms of the whiplash syndrome, and ultimately to my exploration of the somatic syndromes associated with trauma.

I am also indebted to the studies of numerous researchers in the field of trauma. The books and review articles of psychiatrist and traumatologist, Bessel van der Kolk, and his personal advice about this book have been especially helpful. His extensive review articles on the psychobiology of stress and trauma reenactment provided a wealth of background information.

The seminal book, *Affect Development and the Origin of the Self,* by Allan Schore, provided powerful support for concepts of the neurobiology of experience-based development and alteration of brain chemistry and circuitry, a central thesis for this book. Through our personal interaction and his writings, Dr. Schore has been a mentor and a rich source of information.

A recent book on auto accident-related PTSD, *After the Crash,* by psychologists Edward Blanchard and Edward Hickling, validated my own strong impressions that the phenomenon of traumatization accounts for most of the symptoms related to mild-to-moderate motor vehicle accidents (MVAs). This book also underscored the fact that MVAs are a substantial and relatively poorly appreciated cause of societal traumatic stress.

Other individuals who have provided input and help through long discussions about trauma and its meaning include Michael Gismondi,

Jim Grigsby, Melvin Grusing, Marcus Kurek, Joseph Kurtz, Dianne La Tourette, Carol Schneider, Kathleen Shea, Richard Suddath, Sally Thomas, Lynn Waelde, and Gretchen Williams, to name a few.

I am grateful to Michael Scaer for assistance in figure design.

I have learned a great deal from the writings of the many experts in the field of traumatic stress, and am very grateful to them for facilitating my travels in search of knowledge. I could not have even approached this topic without the dedicated help of Connie Cencich-Myers, medical librarian at Boulder Community Hospital. Her tireless assistance in my pursuit of the literature addressing the rapidly emerging field of the psychophysiology and neurobiology of trauma has allowed me to expedite my education and to formulate my own theories of trauma on a sound foundation of knowledge of the literature.

Finally, I perhaps am most grateful to my patients, whose stories, insights, and courage in the face of terrible pain have taught me a great deal of what this book is about. They have taught me that if a physician lets his patients tell him everything they have to say, that physician is likely to know everything there is to know. The many case studies that fill the pages to come are all true and accurate, although names have been changed throughout, and the stories modified to protect anonymity.

Chapter 1

Concepts of Traumatization: The Role of Boundaries

Jane came into my office clearly in a state of distraction and fear. She had been involved in a relatively low-speed auto accident two months before, and instead of improving, she had begun to experience worsening cognitive and emotional symptoms. She had begun to misplace things constantly, had spells of severe physical weakness, had fallen several times, and had developed a stutter. At other times she felt agitated and fearful, and was intolerant of any stimulus, including noises, bright lights, and even simple conversation with family and friends. Even brief exposure to these seemingly minor stimuli produced confusion, anxiety, and ultimately exhaustion. When I examined her, she visibly jumped, and then pulled her arms tightly around herself when I walked around the back of the exam table to examine her spine. When asked, she stated that she felt extremely anxious and uncomfortable when I stood behind her out of her field of vision, even with a female chaperone in the room. Her past social history revealed that she had experienced a physically traumatic rape at age sixteen. She acknowledged that she had always been uncomfortable in situations where she was in a crowd with people behind her that she could not see. In a classroom, a theater, or at a party, she usually positioned herself with her back to the wall.

* * *

The benchmark for psychiatric diagnoses, the *Diagnostic and Statistical Manual of Mental Disorders*, Fourth Edition (DSM-IV), defines trauma as, "The person experienced, witnessed, or was confronted with an event or events that involved actual or threatened death or serious injury, or a threat to the physical integrity of self or others." In addition, trauma requires that "the person's responses involved intense fear, helplessness, or horror"[1] (pp. 427, 428). In earlier editions, the DSM was more vague, defining trauma in part as ". . . a stressful occurrence that is outside the range of usual human experience . . ."[2] (p. 236). The critical change in this definition is the addition to the concept of trauma that involves ". . . threatened death or serious injury." In other words, this concept now implies that trauma is an event or experience that threatens the survival of the individual.

Examples of traumatic events that the DSM-IV lists include ". . . military combat, violent personal assault (sexual assault, physical attack, robbery, mugging), . . . kidnapping, . . . being taken hostage, terrorist attack, torture, POW, natural or man-made disasters, severe MVA's, . . . life threatening illnesses"[1] (p. 424). For children, "developmentally inappropriate sexual experiences without violence" may be traumatic[1] (p. 424). Actually viewing these types of traumatic events or seeing a dead body may be traumatic. Learning about these types of events occurring to a family member or close personal friend also may be defined as trauma[1] (p. 424). When the trauma is inflicted by another person, is especially intense, or the traumatized person is extremely close to the trauma, the severity of traumatization may be especially profound.

These definitions of trauma and its causes are useful, and much more specific than earlier concepts of sources of trauma as representing "stressful events outside the usual range of human experience." However, they still do not approach the basic premise that in all cases, a traumatic experience in its basic sense is one that represents a threat to the very survival of the individual. In this definition, the *meaning* of the event may be as important to the traumatized person as what actually physically happens to that person.

Being kidnapped, mugged, raped, involved in warfare, or in a severe MVA are life-threatening experiences, and therefore potentially traumatizing. Photographs of survivors of tornadoes, floods, or other natural disasters clearly reflect the shock, grief, and suffering associated with shocking and life-threatening natural events. Witnessing a graphically violent event could be perceived as shocking and traumatizing, especially if the event had personal meaning or involved another human being. Childhood trauma is perhaps the easiest to understand, given the intrinsic vulnerability of the developing child to all types of experiences. Even learning secondhand about a severe traumatic event involving a loved one generally is a source of shock to a person. How all of these events may represent a threat to one's survival is less clear unless one considers the concept more carefully.

THE CONCEPT OF BOUNDARIES

We all live in a small and safe world of our own defined by invisible but very real barriers, or boundaries. These boundaries are formed by our collective experiences with the world around us, some of which are positive or rewarding, some negative or punishing. Negative experiences are associated with pain, which may be as obvious as physical discomfort, or as subtle as withdrawal of a reward. Perhaps one of the earliest pains that we are likely to experience is the disapproving frown of our mother to our irritating infantile behavior, producing shame, and creating perhaps the first boundary in the perception of the infant-mother connection. All of our senses—smell, vision, hearing, vestibular input, taste, touch, nociception and proprioception—contribute to the formation of these boundaries that eventually tell us where we as a perceptual whole end, and the rest of the world begins. Our unconscious awareness of these boundaries allows us to move about in the world without literally impacting obstacles that are not part of our own self. As a developing infant and child, we receive positive or negative information from sensory experiences that contribute to our unconscious perception of our safe boundaries. Painful or unpleasant feedback leads us to avoid moving beyond the boundary created by that experience, whereas positive feedback stimulates us to explore that boundary area more. Based on this sensory feedback loop, we are continuously forming and reforming our boundaries based on our continuing life experiences and the sensory messages associated with them. From these experiences, we form a very specific awareness of the safe extent to which we may challenge the world around us. Theoretically, the perceptual concept of our boundaries could be equated at least partly to our sense of self. Logically, the more positive our ongoing life experience is and the more intense the associated positive sensory experience is the more solid our personal sense of boundary will become. The more solid that our boundaries are, the more safe, secure, and effective we will be in dealing with the world outside of us. In many respects, this concept of boundary envisions an almost tangible, physiologically and perceptually based entity.

THE ROLE OF BOUNDARIES IN TRAUMA

How does this discussion of esoteric and invisible boundaries relate to concepts of traumatization and threats to our survival? From our infancy, we identify those objects in our environment that are essential to our survival through the process of boundary definition. Obviously the first persons with whom we identify are our caregivers, particularly our mothers, through maternal-child attunement. From these critical figures in our early childhood milieu, we hopefully receive more rewarding experiences than we ever will receive again in our lives. With our caregivers, we are able to expand our boundaries far beyond our perceived physical selves. Before the sense of shame is inevitably introduced, we are literally without a sense of boundary between ourselves and our maternal caregiver. But the early infancy maternal-child bond is temporary, and boundaries must be formed for survival of the growing child, hence the necessary introduction of shame as a boundary-forming tool. Shame is usually first experienced by the infant in response to its own behavior that is felt to be in excess of acceptable expression by the mother.[3] By means of an initial negative facial expression in response to this behavior, the mother signals displeasure, instilling in the infant its first sense of boundary definition. Nevertheless, in a healthy caregiver and family environment, the growing child will experience a sense of expansive and generous boundaries, where his or her sense of self may range widely and freely without risk of traumatic impact. When the growing child experiences threat, hurt, or shame outside the safe haven of the caregivers, these nurturing individuals are always there to address the hurt, discharge the threat, and in effect rebuild the safe boundary. At the same time, in the interests of survival, a solid sense of where one indeed does impact the rest of the world is instilled in gradual ways through subtle negative maternal feedback. A strong sense of self and of boundaries separating us from the world around us gives us unique resilience to deal with perceived threats to survival, which inevitably impinge upon us in our daily lives. Using this concept of boundary allows us to understand why all of the relatively disparate examples of trauma in the DSM-IV have in common the specific concept of threats to survival.

Violent physical assault in any form needs no rationalization to qualify as a survival-threatening event. The sense of safe separation between the assaulted person and the real world is shattered, especially if associated with physical pain and injury. Although a life-threatening illness presents a less physically tangible assault on one's sense of self, the safe haven of our body is ruptured and redefined. Once again, witnessing a violent event involving life-threatening bodily injury or death may redefine what constitutes a safe boundary for us, may shrink that boundary, and therefore constitute a threat to our survival.

BOUNDARIES AND CHILDHOOD

In a child whose boundaries are evolving, ebbing and flowing with new life experiences, vulnerability to traumatic stress is extreme. In our society, we are taught from infancy by means of word, inference, or simple behavior that our sexual expression constitutes the most private and central part of our self, and therefore represents the most vulnerable zone of our boundary awareness. It is quite reasonable that ". . . developmentally inappropriate sexual experiences without . . . violence . . ." might still constitute a threat to survival of the vulnerable child[1] (p. 424). In addition, the child's caregiver(s) and immediate family provide the child with their intrinsic sense of self, and create their initial sense of safe boundary with the world. Death, critical illness or injury, or even the threat of these events happening to those important individuals clearly represent to the child a threat to his or her own existence. Even in adulthood, the meaning of those individuals in our life remains as it was as a child, and threats to the existence of our former caregivers remain a threat to our survival.

The most devastating form of traumatic stress therefore clearly occurs when caregivers, the intrinsic safe haven, the providers of our basic sense of boundaries, become the existential threat. When the maternal caregiver at times is also the raging and alcoholic abuser, when the loving father is also the source of incest, molestation, or physical abuse, there is no safe haven and no safe boundary between the child and his or her outside world. The child's perception of self is constricted and shrunken, with little residual buffer between what is perceived as a safe, bounded space and the unknowable threats of the external environment. As a result, it takes a much smaller or less intense perceived threat to create traumatic stress for such a child when the source of that threat is a caregiver. In the absence of a generous boundary, the child has lost resilience and the ability to test the world, to take risks in order to establish a healthy sense of self-perception. As this child approaches adulthood, stresses and threats that might be considered trivial tend to assume the proportions of threats to survival. This at least in part contributes to the well-known phenomena of vulnerability to trauma, and of retraumatization in these individuals.

The next line of defense, the next presumably safe line of boundary formation, lies within the expanding network of other members of our human species. As one progresses from less immediate family members, through close friends, neighborhoods, tribes, cultures, religions, and nations, the pivotal importance of these members of our human society to maintain our safe boundary perception gradually diminishes. Eventually human members of other tribes, religions, or nations may represent mortal threats. Nevertheless, those members of the human species apart from our immediate caregivers who are still perceived to be close in their relationship to us represent to a significant degree a source of safe boundary perception. Therefore, traumatization may be especially severe when it is inflicted by any other human being. Trauma resulting from rape, assault, and torture is known to be especially devastating, probably because all of these acts represent a loss of sense of safety or boundary between us and members of our own species.

CONCLUSION

From a conceptual standpoint, then, we are defining trauma, or a traumatic event, as anything that represents a threat to our survival as a human being. The mechanism by which traumatic stress occurs is by impinging upon, or rupturing, that intangible but very real perceptual boundary that separates our safe sense of self from the world around us. Although this, of course, is a theoretical model, it explains why the severity of trauma is worst with experiencing, less with witnessing, and least with learning about it—in other words, the closer the traumatic experience, the worse the damage. The boundary model explains why even lesser degrees of trauma inflicted by another person may be a mortal threat if that person represents a vital resource in the formation of our safe boundaries. Finally, it illustrates the reasons why trauma is most devastating when it comes from persons or events surrounding those persons who are the primary source of our safe boundary formation, our primary caregivers.

We specifically did not address the issue of the person's response to a traumatic event, although as we shall see, that response is critical to the victim's physiological response to that trauma, and its effect on his or her resulting well-being. We do not feel that fear or horror are necessary to the process of traumatization, but concur that helplessness is an intrinsic variable without which traumatization is unlikely to occur. The neurophysiological features of the response to trauma in a state of perceived helplessness forms the thesis for this book. As you will see, the concept of boundaries is also central to that thesis.

Chapter 2

Trauma, Instinct, and the Brain:
The Fight/Flight/Freeze Response

When I was a kid living on the farm, I woke up one morning to a weird sound, almost like a baby crying. I went outside, and in the yard was an opossum, lying there crying and gasping for breath. He had a broken bottle around his neck that was choking him. He must have gotten it stuck around his neck when he was young, and as he grew it eventually began to choke him. So I got a towel and wrapped him in it so he wouldn't bite me, and he went limp and unconscious. I cracked the bottleneck with a hammer, unwrapped him, and he just lay there for a few minutes. Then he began to shake all over on the ground, and after about a minute, got up and staggered off.

This story was told to me by a patient who had been injured in an auto accident, and who had experienced a similar physical event that he had observed in the opossum as a child.

* * *

Over the past century, theories concerning the biological response of the body to acute and chronic stress have developed that have gradually clarified the intricate and interrelated neurophysiological, hormonal, and behavioral events involved in this process. Cannon presented the concept of the sympathetic-adrenal stress response, linking the role of the adrenal medulla and epinephrine to the body's adaptation to emergencies.[1] Selye introduced the theory of a general adaptation syndrome (GAS) in response to prolonged stress, characterized by three phases: alarm, resistance, and exhaustion.[2] His concept addressed not only the acute fight/flight response, but also the sustained effort of the body in the face of ongoing life-threatening stress.

The neural pathways for the acute response to a threat begin with sensory input from various organ systems to the thalamus. This varied information may arise from any of the organs of sensing, including sight, smell, taste, hearing, or kinesthetic and pain sensations. Except for olfaction, which accesses the amygdala directly without traversing the filter of the thalamus, sensory information pertaining to this arousal-based sensory information is routed to the thalamus, from which it is further routed to appropriate areas of the cerebral cortex. Similar information is also sent by the thalamus to the limbic system, particularly the amygdala, the center for memory as it pertains to arousal. The emotional content and meaning of this sensory input are assessed by the right amygdala, which essentially attaches an emotional valence to that information for the purpose of further information and memory processing by the right hippocampus and orbitofrontal cortex.[3] Input via norepinephrine from the locus ceruleus, a part of the reticular activating system, is also provided directly to the amygdala, which further assesses the arousal-based content of this sensory input.[4] The right orbitofrontal cortex organizes cortical and brainstem defensive sensorimotor responses as well as autonomic responses to this threat (see Figure 2.1).

Centers in the hypothalamus related to the brain's arousal system are also activated through orbitofrontal cortical input, and facilitate sympathetic nervous system pathways, leading to the release of epinephrine by the adrenal medulla. Input from the locus ceruleus also triggers activation of the hypothalamic/pituitary/adrenal (HPA) axis (see Figure 2.2). Hypothalamic release of corticotrophic releasing hormone (CRH) triggers release of adrenal corticotrophic hormone (ACTH) by the pituitary, which in turn facilitates release of cortisol by the adrenal cortex. The specific systemic effects of epinephrine include mobilization of glycogen by the liver with increase in blood sugar, vasoconstriction in skin and viscera, vasodilatation in skeletal muscles, and increase in pulse, blood pressure, and cardiac output. Cortisol promotes sodium retention, which results in increased blood volume, and also mobilizes serum lipids and increases blood sugar. It also inhibits ongoing energy-mobilizing effects of epinephrine, inhibits the HPA axis, and provides a modulatory effect on fight/flight activation of these systems. Later effects of cortisol promote sus-

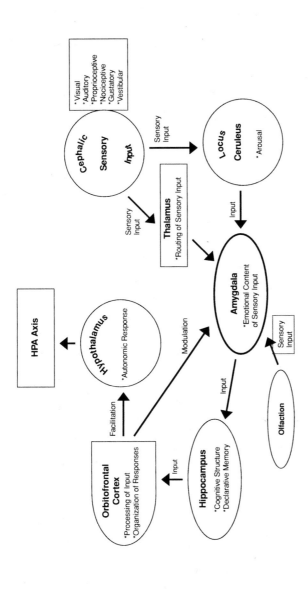

FIGURE 2.1. Theoretical diagram of pathways for arousal and memory mechanisms in the brain in response to a threat. Sensory input is transmitted directly to the brainstem locus ceruleus, and routed through the thalamus except for olfaction, which is transmitted directly to the locus ceruleus and amygdala. Input from these information resources is routed to the right amygdala, where it is evaluated for its emotional content. Related information from the amygdala is then routed to the hippocampus, the center for declarative memory, where a cognitive structure for the information is developed. This information is then transmitted to the right orbitofrontal cortex where it is processed, and a behavioral and autonomic response to the threat is organized.

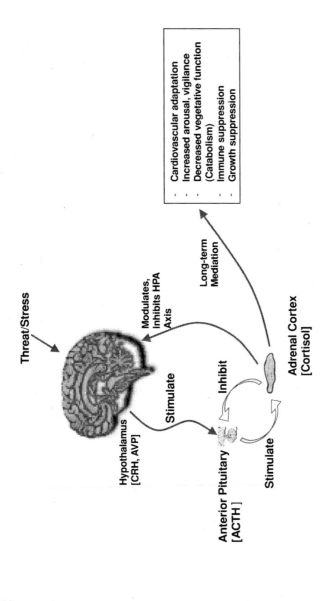

FIGURE 2.2. Hypothalamic/pituitary/adrenal axis. Sensory input signaling stress or threat (see Figure 2.1) activates the hypothalamus, triggering release of corticotropin-releasing hormone (CRH) and arginine vasopressin (AVP). These promote release of cortisol from adrenal medulla. Cortisol inhibits further release of ACTH, modulates the basic noradrenergic arousal response, and mediates the long-term stress adaptation response to stress.

12

tained cardiovascular stability in the face of ongoing stress and prevent circulatory collapse at the expense of short-term sacrifice of energy storage and diffuse tissue injury or catabolism. Some researchers also feel that the more slowly acting cortisol effect may act to facilitate avoidance conditioning in response to ongoing stress.[5]

BRAIN RESPONSES TO STRESS

Central nervous system effects triggered by release of norepinephrine include increased alertness and focus, immediate facilitation of short-term memory, pupillary dilatation and ocular divergence, as well as increased skeletal muscle tone. The immediate effects of epinephrine and norepinephrine prepare the organism for the high level neuromuscular activity required for ensuring survival in the face of threat—the fight/flight response. These effects promote short-term preparation of the brain for intense alertness, and the neuromuscular and cardiovascular systems for high level short-term skeletal muscle activity and energy expenditure. Activation of the fight/flight response, of course, may be triggered by excitement as well as by threat. The basic physiological response of the prey in response to threat is mirrored by that of the predator as it prepares for attack. Pregame jitters, stage fright, sexual arousal, and the thrill of the roller coaster ride all reflect the physical sensations associated with arousal in the face of threat. What separates the experience of the fight/flight response from that of anticipatory excitement, of course, is the *meaning* of the event to the participant. This piece of information processing takes place in the hippocampus (comparison of new information with past associative memories), and the orbitofrontal cortex (problem solving and planning).[4] Whether the animal, or human, then assumes the role of predator or prey based on this higher level cognitive process, the end result of epinephrine-based arousal is similar—the initiation of intense muscular activity and exertion. Excitatory neurotransmitters and hormones fuel both the flight of the prey and the attack of the predator, initiating a high-level energy expenditure response by the neuromuscular system. In the pecking order of eating and being eaten throughout the animal kingdom, many species operate both as prey and predator, and mobilize epinephrine at both ends of the spectrum. Epinephrine is an equal opportunity energizer, and whether the weasel is catching a mouse, or being caught by a hawk, the initial physiological effects of both predation and defense are similar in many respects, and contribute to the function of resisting, escaping, or attacking. Very soon, however, the *meaning* of the arousal sequence assumes an important role in subsequent neurohumoral events. Mason has introduced the role of "psychological" meaning into the stress response equation, disputing Selye's avoidance of cognitive mediation of the stress response. Under Mason's concepts, a more complex interaction of cortical/hypothalamic/pituitary circuitry is involved in the stress response, and allows for a broader range of behavioral response to threat or arousal. Thus, the later neurohormonal events of predation and defense diverge and lead to quite different behavioral and physiological sequences.[6]

Other brain neurotransmitter systems also contribute to the effectiveness of the fight/flight response. Norepinephrine, as we have noted, facilitates alerting mechanisms and transmission of messages throughout the central sympathetic pathways. Endorphins, the brain's pain-modulating neurotransmitters, are also released, accounting for the well-documented increased pain threshold in acute arousal.[7,8] The obvious function served by endorphins includes blunting of pain reflexes and inhibition of conscious and unconscious self-protective responses that might interfere with effective survival behavior. For example, with the aid of the analgesic effects of endorphins released with fight/flight arousal, the injured soldier is able to complete the physical activity necessary for his survival without the interference of debilitating pain.

Release of endorphins as part of arousal also has interesting implications concerning brain reward mechanisms in human behavior. Since arousal related to predation or excitement is also linked to endorphin release, it is easy to appreciate the reward involved in high-risk recreational activities associated with the "adrenaline rush," since this experience also involves endorphinergic reward. Risk-taking thrills seem unique to the human species, and it is clear that certain personality traits may predispose to this behavior. There is even some evidence that this trait may be apparent in childhood. At any rate, one does not see weasels jumping into the talons of hawks just to experience the thrill of the wild ride. Once again, the meaning of the event that triggers the relatively stereotyped initial neurohumoral contributions to the fight/flight response likely has a marked effect on later neurohumoral events and behaviors. Risk-taking and the human element related to reward from endorphins in arousal may well contribute to the peculiar tendency for trauma reenactment in PTSD, as we shall explore in Chapter 7.

FIGHTING, FLEEING, OR FREEZING

Animals and humans cycle in and out of varying states of arousal many times a day in response to thousands of widely varying stimuli. This cycle takes place between the *ergotropic,* or energy spending activity of the sympathetic nervous system, and the *trophotropic,* or energy storing activity of the parasympathetic nervous system.[9] The main effects of activation of the parasympathetic nervous system, mediated by the neurotransmitter acetylcholine, include slowing of the heart, lowering the blood pressure, shunting of blood away from the muscles and to the abdominal viscera, activation of the digestive process, and storage of nutrients. It is also the state in which acquisition of information and operation of declarative memory in storage of facts and events best takes place, in that high levels of norepinephrine may interfere with certain types of memory storage.[10] Although the parasympathetic nervous system is relatively inactivated in arousal, it does play a role in the freeze, or immobility response, the third and least understood or appreciated part of the fight/flight/freeze sequence.

The Animal Model

Those of us fascinated by animal behavior in the wild love to watch shows on TV devoted to observations of animals in this setting. Many of these TV specials relate to the prey/predator experience, and sometimes display this in graphic and even grisly detail, at least to our civilized eye. If one closely watches the details of pursuit of the prey by the predator, one will see that the fleeing prey will often collapse and become limp even before being seized by the predator. An example is a film that I saw involving a gazelle pursued and run to the ground by a cheetah. At the moment that the cheetah caught the gazelle, it struck the gazelle lightly on the flank, at which point the gazelle collapsed and lay inert on the ground in the freeze or immobility response. In another example, after fighting off a pride of lions for over half an hour, the lone water buffalo was knocked off his feet, at which point he became limp, immobile, and frozen. In other words, when fleeing and fighting are no longer physically possible, and the prey animal is in a state of helplessness, it will frequently enter the freeze, or immobility state, a totally instinctual and unconscious reflex. This behavior is common in most species including insects, reptiles, birds, and mammals. Since most such reflexes have evolved as a means of perpetuating the species, the freeze response clearly is of critical importance for survival. In a surprising number of cases, the attack of the predator may be fueled by the convenient presence of the prey rather than by hunger, in which case the freeze response of the prey may abort the instinctive attack of the predator and result in survival of the prey. The freeze response mimics death, sometimes fooling the predator enough to leave the scene of her "kill" and gather her offspring without delivering the tooth and claw coup de grâce, thereby allowing the prey to recover and escape, as in "playing possum." In addition, the freeze response, analogous at least in part to dissociation in humans, is associated with additional release of endorphins, rendering the animal relatively analgesic (see Chapter 8). Whether this analgesia has survival value, or is a gift from a greater Being to prevent a painful death is open to debate. Another purpose of freeze analgesia may be to inhibit self-ministering behavior, such as wound licking, which would impede escape of the prey animal in the case of arousal from the freeze.

The basic laboratory model of the freeze response utilizes the method of inescapable shock (IS).[11] Although acute IS in the previously unexposed animal initially induces a state of acute arousal and defensive postures, subsequent IS elicits a consistent freeze in the face of manifest helplessness. In escapable shock (ES), the animal will quickly discover the means of escape through trial and error, and never experience a freeze. By definition, that option does not exist in IS. Trial and error escape techniques are to no avail, and in the face of continued shock/threat in the face of helplessness, the animal will eventually freeze. Animals who have experienced IS and freezing sufficiently in the past will continue to exhibit passive immobility and continued freeze in the face of repetitive IS, even if presented with a new possibility of escape.[12] They seem to have lost their ability to problem-solve and learn, having faced shock in the past without means of escape. In addition, animals exposed to several episodes of IS linked in time with neutral stimuli will begin to exhibit freezing in the face of the neutral conditioned stimuli presented independently.[13] A freeze response triggered by a traumatic event may become linked to ambient environmental cues through conditioning. These environmental cues, although intrinsically benign, may then serve as traumatic stimuli. Finally, attempts to break through freezing from IS through shock as a punishing stimulus result in relative increase in freeze behavior rather than triggering escape behavior.[14] These findings therefore suggest that repetitive exposure to IS seems to impair basic storage of memory and information; to condition the freeze response to benign but trauma-related cues; and to assure that freezing will eventually follow trauma even if escape is feasible. Comparison of these animal behaviors has led van der Kolk and colleagues to postulate that the psychophysiological disorder of post-traumatic stress disorder (PTSD) may have a biological model in the response of animals to IS.[15] Such observations have also led Nijenhuis, Vanderlinden, and Spinhoven to draw a parallel between animal defensive traits that are triggered by severe life threat, such as freezing, and the characteristics of dissociative states in patients with major dissociation.[16]

Assumption of the immobility response is associated with a dramatic change in the state of autonomic equilibrium, along with the release of endogenous opioids. The racing heart slows to a crawl, blood pressure drops precipitously, tense muscles collapse and become still as a result of the assumption of an apparent enforced vegetative state. The focused and alert mind becomes numb and dissociated, at least in part due to high levels of endorphins. Memory access and storage are impaired, and amnesia may be expected for at least some of the events occurring during the freeze. The frozen animal is in a state of suspended animation, with high levels of parasympathetic and endorphinergic activity.[17] The physiology of the freeze response in essence involves a state of high-level parasympathetic tone, with additional residuals of the preceding state of high sympathetic arousal, a distinct state of departure from the usual homeostatic equilibrium between sympathetic and parasympathetic systems.

The Freeze Discharge

In most cases, the frozen prey animal does not need to deal with the presumably unhealthy state of the freeze response—it becomes another animal's meal. High levels of epinephrine, endorphins, and acetylcholine apparently do not affect taste. Fortunately, high levels of endorphins render the animal relatively analgesic. In some cases, however, the frozen prey animal survives the period of immobility without being killed. Subsequent events in this case are of critical importance to the thesis of this book. In virtually all such instances, the animal will arouse and begin to tremble. This may be as imperceptible as a shudder, or as dramatic as a grand mal seizure. In some cases analyzed by slow motion video, the trembling will resemble the last act of the animal before freezing—the act of running. The animal's behavior at times seems to resemble an unconscious attempt to complete the act of survival, as if the last protective motor or muscular activity is locked in unconscious procedural memory and needs to be released, or completed, perhaps as a means of "discharging" retained autonomic energy. At the same time, the animal may perspire. This motor and autonomic response may persist for several minutes, and is usually terminated by a series of deep, sighing breaths. The animal at this point will usually arouse fully, regain its feet, often stagger a bit, shake itself, and then run off, apparently none the worse for its life-threatening experience. Long-term observations of such animals do not seem to show any harmful effects on behavior, health, or other measures of survival. It would appear from these observations that animals in the wild possibly possess an instinctual means of dissipating autonomic activity stored and accumulated in the freeze response.[18]

This remarkable phenomenon may occur in a much more subtle fashion, and may take place many times a day in the life of a prey animal. The gazelle may arouse to the scent of predators on many occasions, manifesting and alerting response with tensing of muscles, and with scanning movements of the head and eyes, an instinctual behavior called orientation common to all species. The perceived absence of threat is usually then followed by return to the calm grazing state, but usually only after a slight muscular shudder or trembling.[18] The bird that inadvertently flies into a window and is stunned will often remain immobile when picked up by the concerned homeowner and cradled in her hand. When set down on the ground, it will frequently arouse, shake, or tremble, and then fly away, having effectively discharged the stored autonomic energy of its freeze, which probably occurred as much because of handling by the "predator" as by the impact with the window. A patient told me a story about saving a caged pet rabbit from a burning house. The rabbit appeared limp, unresponsive, and supposedly dead when found by the homeowner. Suddenly the rabbit "went into convulsions," after which it aroused and then appeared to be normal. What the patient interpreted as an episode of smoke inhalation in a rabbit was clearly a freeze response, with a healthy and life-affirming discharge of retained autonomic energy through a sterotyped neuromuscular reflex response that, in fact, may have represented completion of the truncated act of flight.

The Human Anomaly

Very little literature addresses the freeze response in the human species. Even in the case of overwhelming threat and trauma, it is rare for a human being to actually collapse and appear unconscious without physical injury. Although some people will be shaky and tremulous after a shocking event, they seldom pursue the relatively stereotyped behavior seen in animals. Rather, they will frequently relate that they felt as if they were "in shock." This is often related as a sense of detachment, numbness, and even confusion. Time often seems to stand still. Some patients report that they feel as if they are detached and removed from their body, occasionally reporting the events of the trauma as if they were seeing them as a third person. Although some will relate that they were "full of adrenaline," many report the sensation as one of remarkable calm. Although serious injuries may have occurred, pain is usually not intense during this period, an event consistent with the role of endorphins in the freeze response. Psychologists commonly refer to this phenomenon as dissociation, which is defined as "An unconscious process by which a group of mental processes is separated from the rest of the thinking processes, resulting in an independent functioning of these processes and a loss of the usual relationships; for example, a separation of affect from cognition."[19] Dissociation very probably constitutes a major element of the freeze response, and people who report symptoms of shock and numbness after a traumatic event, and exhibit symptoms of dissociation, are actually in the freeze response at the time. In fact many of the posttraumatic symptoms that occur often for years after the unresolved trauma are characteristic of dissociation, or recurrence of the symptoms of freezing.

The salient point here is that human beings seem to recover from this state of shock without any of the physical and muscular activity observed in animals as they recover from the act of freezing after a threat. One seldom sees victims of an acute traumatic event falling to the ground, shaking, trembling, or sweating, and recovering with a period of slow, heavy breathing. One is tempted to consider this response to be a positive adaptation to basic animal behavior as a result of the evolving frontal neocortex which allows us to think, problem solve, and plan without the tyranny of primitive instinct. There is a real concern, however, that this apparent lack of discharge of autonomic energy after the occurrence of freezing in the human species may indeed not be a functional adaptive mechanism. Instead, it may represent a dangerous suppression of instinctual behavior, resulting in the imprinting of the traumatic experience in unconscious memory and arousal systems of the brain.

Acculturation of the human species has resulted in an increasing pattern of urban living in closely confined habitats that intrinsically may inhibit the instinctual capability to flee or defend oneself under threat. This in turn may instill a state of helplessness, predisposing to the freeze response in humans under threat. This same state of intense proximity and cultural interdependence may also act to inhibit the natural discharge of autonomic freeze energy in such cases.

An answer to this dilemma may lie in observation of animal behavior. Levine describes a conversation that he had with African gamekeepers.[18] When captured, animals commonly enter a freeze, or immobility, response. After release, they will usually go through a form of behavior typical of the freeze discharge described above. If they do not go through a period of shaking, however, they will usually die after release into the wild. This fact might lead one to speculate that retaining the tremendous autonomic energy of the fight/flight/freeze response in the bodies and central nervous systems of these animals reduces their capacity to adapt to the threats and demands of existence in the wild. Clearly, self-protective behavior in animals is likely to be inhibited by behavior analogous to a state of intermittent dissociation in humans. In fact, there is also evidence that freeze discharge may also be inhibited in animals chronically maintained in captivity, such as domesticated and laboratory animals, as well as residents of zoos and circuses. Indeed, early studies of the stress response in laboratory animals were limited by the intrinsic arousal associated with handling, leading to the freeze response, and subsequent "experimental neurosis."

Theoretical models of kindling as a likely neurophysiological event in the development of symptoms of PTSD after a traumatizing experience are presented in Chapter 4. The self-perpetuated circuitry involved in kindling is remarkably compatible with absence of discharge of the defensive sensorimotor sequence of behavior that precedes the freeze or immobility response. Retention in procedural memory of this experience may serve as a recurrent internal cue for recurrent arousal patterns, alternating with numbing and dissociation, constituting the basically bipolar and self-perpetuating nature of PTSD. Until that act of flight or self defense has been completed, therefore, the "survival brain" may continue to perceive that the threat continues to exist, and is unable to relegate it to memory as a past experience.

CONCLUSION

The theory that human traumatization has its roots in inhibition of the freeze discharge after surviving a mortal threat has important implications for treatment of physical and emotional disorders in victims of trauma. The neurophysiological and neurohormonal events involved in the fight/flight/freeze response clearly have profound effects on all organ systems of the body. I believe that the effects of the unresolved freeze response on the body and brain have important implications for concepts and treatment of human disease. The truncated freeze discharge appears to be the physiological event that initiates the central nervous system changes leading the post-traumatic stress disorder. Many of those chronic diseases that seem to be the most common, and which the field of allopathic medicine has been most ineffective in treating, may well have their roots in the insidious systemic effects of traumatization. In fact, I believe that the most common complaint in current medical practice, that of persistent and unexplained chronic pain, has its roots in the persistent changes in brain circuitry associated with unresolved traumatization, and the continued tendency for dissociation to occur in the face of stress or threat. As we have noted, the pattern of defensive and protective movement at the time of a traumatic event is stored in procedural memory for the purpose of adaptation to future related threat, and incorporated in regional neuromuscular detail into the kindled cycle of trauma. By the same token, the somesthetic and nociceptive thalamic input associated with the same threat is stored in conditioned procedural memory, leading to perpetuation of the pain experience as a dysfunctional survival tool. These concepts will be explored in more detail in Chapter 8.

As noted earlier, the bulk of my experience in human trauma is in MVA-related injuries, and the majority of these patients have the diagnosis of whiplash. The beauty of using the whiplash syndrome as a model for trauma is the fact that patients who have experienced this injury routinely present with a startlingly similar cluster of symptoms, many of which defy logical medical explanation. As you will see, however, all of these varied and multisystemic symptoms are remarkably and logically explainable when viewed from the model of an aborted freeze discharge and its neurophysiological and behavioral implications, in the absence of tangible physical injury. Whiplash and its associated symptom complex represent a uniquely graphic depiction of the somatic consequences of traumatization when viewed as a function of a truncated freeze discharge.

Chapter 3

The Whiplash Syndrome I:
Symptoms in Search of a Meaning

THE HISTORY OF WHIPLASH

Recognized for over 100 years, criticized, analyzed, debated, defended, debunked, and generally misunderstood, the complex group of symptoms that follow velocity-related injuries in vehicles of conveyance continues to defy medical scientific explanation. With the advent of the railroad in the nineteenth century, a group of symptoms of chronic neck and back pain associated with severe emotional disturbance was described in association with train accidents. It was generally called "Railroad Spine," and was placed in the category of psychoneuroses.[1] With the invention of the automobile, reports of persisting neck pain after MVAs began to appear as early as 1919.[2] The noted American author, Mark Twain, described the physical properties producing whiplash when he described the skills of his hero, Huckleberry Finn, in beheading snakes by snapping them like a whip. The first use of the term "whiplash" in medicine occurred in an article in 1945.[3] In 1953, Gay and Abbott described the condition of "whiplash" in detail. They clearly stated the dilemma that has continued to plague physicians, patients, and insurance companies: "Characteristically, these patients were more disabled and remained handicapped for longer periods than was anticipated, considering the mild character of the accident."[4] Severy and colleagues further amplified this dilemma in their 1955 study, observing, ". . . unlike most injury-producing accidents, there is generally no visible sign of injury for the rear-end collision victim."[5] Because of this remarkable discrepancy in many whiplash patients, some doctors have gone to great lengths to discredit the concept that actual spinal injury could occur at speeds of 10 mph or less. Some have tested the forces of "perturbations of daily living," such as plopping into a chair, slapping on the back, and jumping off a step, and have found forces comparable to a low velocity MVA.[6] Other physicians have taken the wide spectrum of symptoms occurring after a whiplash in addition to neck pain, and concluded that only compensation neurosis or other emotional factors could cause such a diversity of physical complaints.[7]

THE CLINICAL SYNDROME

Patients suffering from even a minor to moderate velocity rear-end MVA often suffer from a confusing variety of symptoms. Not only do they have the typical complaints of head pain and neck stiffness, they also often complain of emotional symptoms, depression, and anxiety. Neurological complaints are common, ranging from dizziness and vertigo, blurred vision, fainting spells, and balance difficulties to remarkable problems with thinking, concentration, and memory. Rather than making a steady recovery as with a comparable sports-related accident, whiplash patients often pursue a slow, unpredictable course, often taking several years to improve, with episodic periods of worsening. Long-term studies in whiplash patients in general show that a majority (70 to 80 percent) had returned to normal activities in six months.[8, 9, 10] On the other hand, in other studies, persistent chronic pain has been noted in 18 percent at three years,[11] and up to 40 percent at eight to ten years.[12] It is not surprising that certain segments of the insurance, legal, and medical communities express skepticism concerning the validity of many whiplash symptoms.

PHYSICAL FORCES
AND STRUCTURAL INJURY

Physicians who sincerely believe in the validity of whiplash as a physical injury have gone to great lengths to prove the validity of this syndrome by exhaustively analyzing the forces brought to bear on the body in an MVA.[5,13,14,15] To their credit, they have shown that the forces on the head itself are three to four times greater than on the body with a sudden change in velocity, due to the pendular effect produced by the weight of the head supported by the stalk-like neck. Based on the laws of inertia, we know that a body of mass tends to resist movement when a force is applied to it. As a result, if a car is hit from behind and rapidly moved forward, the logical conclusion for years has been that the head will tend to resist movement, and therefore move backward in relation to the car. As the car then slows, the head will then rebound forward. Interestingly, most whiplash patients only recall the forward movement of their head.

Video reenactment of crash dummies in a whiplash surprisingly reveals that the backward and forward movement of the head is much less than was thought. In fact, the initial movement of the body is backward, as expected, but because of relatively greater inertia of the ten-pound head, it will not move backward as quickly as the body, and will therefore assume a temporary position of flexion relative to the body. The initial head movement, in fact, is actually flexion of the chin, followed by the head moving up and slightly backward, followed by a rebound forward move. These studies suggest that a violent "whiplash" of the head backward and forward is probably less than was previously thought.[16] Despite this finding, the diagnosis almost always given to the neck pain after whiplash is "cervical strain." Stretching and tearing of the ligaments of the jaw joints and the facet joints of the cervical spine, damage and rupture of the intervertebral discs, and compression of cervical nerve roots have all been attributed to these forces.[17,18] Acute cervical disc syndrome with radiculopathy, however, is a rare occurrence after whiplash.[19]

Other velocity-related injuries attributed to whiplash include minor traumatic brain injury with postconcussion syndrome. Shearing of axons related to rapid change in velocity of the semifluid brain is the generally accepted mode of damage to the brain.[19] This injury leads to a specific spectrum of cognitive symptoms, as well as vestibular and often visual complaints.[20,21] This entire spectrum of injuries has been based on theories dependent on at least a minimum force applied to the body. Despite numerous attempts at analysis, however, the complexity of automobile impacts makes accurate force determinations extremely difficult.

At impact speeds of 5 mph or less, a small cluster of patients present with the full-blown syndrome described above, making a justification for physical injury as a basis for the symptoms even more difficult. Perhaps the most remarkable fact is that the symptoms of the whiplash syndrome, regardless of the speed and velocity changes of the accident, are remarkably similar from patient to patient, a fact that has justified the classification of whiplash as a syndrome. These symptoms have all been well documented in the medical literature, in those references noted previously and in others.

THE PATHOPHYSIOLOGY OF WHIPLASH

Physicians and chiropractors who believe that whiplash is a legitimate and quite real set of injuries generally believe that neck pain during the early period after a whiplash is due to tearing and stretching of the cervical ligaments. Ligamentous and other soft tissue healing is generally considered to occur after about six to eight weeks. Other discrepancies also pose a challenge to the concept of prolonged cervical pain related to ligamentous injury in whiplash. The remarkably persistent pain and disability seen in many whiplash patients is seldom seen in recreational activities or sports where the individual is subjected to velocity forces of severity comparable to low to medium velocity MVAs.

Professional racecar drivers throughout relatively long careers are usually subjected to similar forces several times in accidents involving impact, but seldom end their careers because of disabling pain. Cervical injuries in sports involving contact, especially football, are relatively common and occasionally neurologically catastrophic. Chronic disabling cervical pain from ligamentous injuries, however, is rare. Football as a sport would be impossible if persistent cervical pain occurred commonly at impact speeds or change of velocities of 5 to 10 mph.

Myofascial Pain

Much of the neck and shoulder pain seen after six to eight weeks after an MVA is believed to be attributable to myofascial pain. Myofascial pain, of course, is a common condition seen in many types of injuries, and under conditions of life stress. In whiplash, it may persist for months and even years. Even after it subsides, it may recur in the same muscle groups with uncanny persistence with ordinary life stress. I have had the opportunity to follow a few patients over periods of fifteen years with up to three MVAs during that time. Even after the third accident, patterns of myofascial pain, spasm, and trigger points related to the first accident continue to be selectively apparent.

Earlier called fibrositis or myofibrositis, myofascial pain was described by a number of researchers in the late nineteenth century and the early 1900s.[22,23,24] From its earliest descriptions, it has generally been attributed to a sudden violent strain of muscles, ligaments, or tendons, or in some cases to extended overuse of the musculotendinous unit. Clinical features have typically involved the description of tender areas in muscles that contain isolated taut bands of muscle fibers. Within these taut bands one can detect palpable hardness of a small area that is exquisitely painful. When compressed, these areas of unique tenderness refer pain to a usually predictable distant site based on which muscle was being palpated. These painful points were first designated as trigger points, and the name myofascial pain was applied to the condition in 1952.[25] Over the years, clinicians have discovered that injecting saline or local anesthetic into these trigger points not only would consistently produce predictable referred pain, but often would "turn off" the trigger point and associated muscle pain. Autonomic characteristics of trigger points include vasoconstriction, sweating and increased electrodermal response, pilomotor activity, and dermatographia.

Early biopsies of trigger points reveal subtle changes in mitochondria and ATP, with mucopolysaccharide deposition and sarcolemmal disruption, findings suggestive of a dystrophic process, perhaps related to increased metabolic demand in the face of reduced circulation.[26] Many of these findings have not been reproduced in subsequent studies, however.

Theories of causation include, among others, a sarcolemmal energy crisis,[27] a dysfunctional muscle spindle,[28] a dysfunctional extrafusal motor endplate,[28,29] dysfunction in the gamma motoneuron circuitry,[30] and a sustained positive feedback loop from muscle spindle and joint capsule proprioceptors to the cerebellum, basal ganglia, and spinal cord.[31] Myofascial pain appears to be a chronic, self-perpetuating condition that is remarkably resistant to treatment, is often regionally specific, and in some cases may last indefinitely.

Thoracic Outlet Syndrome

With prolonged myofascial pain involving the neck and shoulders, the head will usually be pulled forward, and the shoulders protracted and elevated. The patient usually is acutely aware of this posture but is unable to correct it consciously. The resulting postural deformity results in narrowing of the space bounded by the clavicle, the scapula, and first few ribs—i.e., the thoracic outlet—leading to a postural or myofascial thoracic outlet syndrome (TOS). The brachial plexus, subclavian arteries, and veins pass through this space, and narrowing the space compresses these structures. The softest, most compressible structures are the veins that carry cooler, deoxygenated blood back to the heart. One theory is that myofascial TOS results from relative venous congestion caused by impaired venous return related to postural changes. This in turn causes coolness and mild edema of the hand, pain in the arm, and numbness of the hand due to relative hypoxia of muscles and nerves of the arm. The sensory examination in these cases usually reflects mild hypesthesia in a glove distribution to pin prick because the numbness is circulatory, not neurogenic. Since this is an intermittent phenomenon, objective documentation of impaired venous return has not been well documented.

Another theory attributes TOS in whiplash to myofascial involvement of the scalene muscles that form one border of the TOS. Shortening and spasm of the scalene muscles might not only narrow the available space by elevating the first two ribs, but also might cause referred pain and numbness to the hand from scalene trigger points.[32] Paresthesia of the hand in whiplash are unfortunately often confused with a cervical radiculopathy or carpal tunnel syndrome. If such patients are found to have a coincidental and unrelated bulging disc on their MRI, they may be subjected to needless surgery.

Piriformis Syndrome

Low back myofascial pain is also common, often affecting the region of the sacroiliac joints, where the sacral base of the spine rests in a V-shaped notch in the pelvis. It also commonly affects the piriformis muscle, a muscle originating on the sacrum, and inserting on the greater tuberosity of the femur. The function of the piriformis is to externally rotate the femur, and to tighten the pelvic floor, as in the Kegel maneuver. The piriformis muscle is usually pierced by the sciatic nerve on its way from the lumbar spine through the pelvic outlet and down the back of the leg. Spasm and shortening of the piriformis muscle may compress the sciatic nerve causing sciatica. This sciatica, unlike lumbosacral radicular pain, therefore encompasses referral patterns of both the L-5 and S-1 nerve roots. Resulting sciatica is associated with numbness or paresthesia in the distribution of these roots, but with no motor symptoms or loss of the Achilles reflex. Although the piriformis syndrome frequently responds to physical therapy, the patient may be at risk for an unnecessary operation if the MRI of the lumbar spine happens to show a coincidental bulging disc and the surgeon fails to detect the subtle elements of the syndrome. A unique feature of the piriformis syndrome in women is presented in Chapter 11.

Tempormandibular Joint Syndrome

Myofascial pain may affect the temporalis and masseter muscles of the jaw, causing jaw and tooth pain, headaches, a feeling of congestion in the ear, and occasionally tinnitus (the TMJ lies immediately in front of the middle ear, semicircular canals, and cochlea). One theory relates postwhiplash TMJ dysfunction to traumatic anterior dislocation of the joint disc cartilage during the moment of neck hyperextension at which point the mandible is anteriorly dislocated due to abnormal jaw opening. The posteriorly attached disc ligament is stretched, leading to laxity and recurrent anterior disc displacement.[33,34] The exact etiology of whiplash-related TMJ syndrome where no actual blow to the jaw occurred, however, remains unknown. Nevertheless, bruxing, or unconscious gritting or clenching of the teeth, is a well-known symptom in whiplash-related TMJ syndrome, often leading to myofascial pain involving the muscle of mastication. Myofascial pain is a major source of much of the pain that persists in whiplash-related TMJ syndrome.

Minor Traumatic Brain Injury

Impairment of cognition after a whiplash is usually attributed to minor traumatic brain injury, or concussion. Documentation of the loss of consciousness formerly was a requirement to establish this diagnosis. It is now felt that any *alteration* of consciousness, such as stunning or confusion at the time of the injury, is adequate to diagnose minor traumatic brain injury in the presence of other criteria.[35] The mechanism of minor traumatic brain injury is thought to be the tearing or stretching of axons (axonal shearing) as a result of forces related to excessive relative changes in velocity of the head during the acceleration/deceleration of the head during the movement of whiplash.[19,36] Studies have shown that actual head impact is not necessary to cause axonal shearing.[37,38] Specific cognitive symptoms seem to be fairly similar and reproducible from patient to patient.

Perhaps the most consistent area of impairment is in speed of information processing.[38] Specific impairment in complex versus simple reaction time,[39] and in multiple measures of divided attention[40] reflects typical problems with multitask performance and complex attention in mildly head injured patients. Short-term memory measures may also reflect impairment.[38] Subjective cognitive complaints in MVA victims usually involve distractibility, unpredictable impairment of short-term memory, and inability to concentrate. Ambient noise may prevent patients from engaging in a conversation due to distraction. They will forget events, appointments, and things they have said to other people. Frequently they will block on words, names or items of familiar information, including overlearned material such as phone numbers and names of acquaintances. When carefully analyzed, most of their cognitive symptoms may be attributable to slowing of information processing and impaired divided attention.

One of the most persistent and debilitating symptoms is that of profound and pervasive fatigue, both cognitive and physical. With ongoing cognitive demands, patients will "shut down," and be unable to continue with high level or sometimes even routine cognitive activity. Usually this fatigue will begin in midafternoon and prevent any further activity for the rest of the day. Physical exhaustion will usually accompany this, even in the absence of physical activity. Fatigue in minor brain injury is generally combined with other diverse elements of the postconcussion syndrome, but is poorly understood.[41]

Neurological Symptoms

Neurological symptoms involving the eyes and sense of balance are also common. Many whiplash patients complain of difficulty focusing, especially with rapid shift of focus, or with close vision. Examination usually reveals that they have abnormal saccadic and slow tracking movements, binocular dysfunction, and convergence insufficiency.[21] Fluctuating monocular refractive errors are also common. All of these findings are usually attributed to minor brain injury and may be associated with substantial reading difficulty.[21] Patients also experience lightheadedness when they arise quickly due to orthostatic hypotension. Vertigo with neck extension or even rotational movements of the head is common, although complaints of dizziness are usually more vague and difficult to define. This symptom has most commonly been attributed to "cervical vertigo," felt to be caused by aberrant proprioceptive afferent input from positional proprioceptors in the cervical and lumbar regions, or by cervical autonomic dysfunction.[42] Vestibular symptoms also are usually attributed to a concussion of the inner ear, a perilymphatic fistula, or a displaced otolith, but may also be felt to be a reflection of minor brain injury.[20,43] Tinnitus, often unilateral, is also experienced, usually with normal audiograms. At times tinnitus may be attributable to unilateral TMJ syndrome, presumably related to edema of the joint and its proximity to the inner ear.[18]

Emotional Symptoms

Finally, emotional symptoms appear in most whiplash victims. For several weeks they may feel numb or detached, but usually they eventually will experience the onset of anxiety and irritability. Associated with this they may experience anxiety specific to automobile travel, especially when a passenger. This may progress to actual panic attacks when other cars drive too closely, approach rapidly behind them, or when the victims drive by the scene of their accident. Actual visual flashbacks of the accident may be experienced. Repeated intrusive thoughts of the accident may interrupt their train of thought. They may begin to feel jittery, tense, and hypervigilant. Exaggerated startle responses to loud noises may occur. Bright lights and loud or unpleasant noises may become intolerable and cause anxiety and "overload." They may begin to awaken at night in a state of alertness or anxiety, sometimes with racing pulse and cold sweat. Nightmares of the accident may periodically awaken them. If enough of these symptoms appear, they will be diagnosed as suffering from post-traumatic stress disorder (PTSD), although many patients will have only a few of these symptoms.[44] Finally, as all of their symptoms persist, they may develop apathy, loss of interest in eating, decline in libido, and a sense of hopelessness, leading to a diagnosis of depression. The sleep disturbance may become one of repetitive awakening with difficulty falling back to sleep. As emotional symptoms appear, many physicians will begin to attribute most or all of their symptoms to psychological causes.[45]

CONCLUSION

In this conceptual model of the whiplash injury, symptoms are attributed to injuries to ligaments and muscles, the notorious and controversial concept of "soft tissue injuries." In other types of soft tissue injuries in which muscles and ligaments are torn, the pain is immediate and severe, associated with swelling of muscles and joints and marked local tenderness. In whiplash, the severe pain usually appears after a delay of several hours, and at times may be delayed by days.

Recovery in other types of soft tissue injuries may be slow, but is usually steady and predictable. In these injuries, symptoms may fluctuate with use of the affected joint, but do not worsen with incidental life stress, as does the spinal myofascial pain of whiplash. Recovery from myofascial pain after an MVA therefore defies the usual medical explanations for soft tissue injuries that occur in other circumstances.

In this model, the cognitive and intellectual problems after an MVA are attributed to axonal shearing as part of a velocity-based cerebral concussion. The entire concept of "postconcussion syndrome" includes many of the other emotional and neurological symptoms already described. These include dizziness, headache, blurred vision, irritability, and sleep disturbance. In addition, all of these symptoms are believed to be due to injury to the brain and the tissues of the head. Postconcussion syndrome, however, tends to follow minor brain injury much more often than more severe brain injury, in which there has been prolonged loss of consciousness for more than twenty-four hours, no memory of the injury, or even brain surgery. Indeed, some studies suggest that the long-term disability after six to twelve months post accident is greater in mild concussion than in moderate brain injury where the patient does not remember the accident.[46] Once again, the neurological problems following a whiplash often are dramatically out of proportion to the severity of the injury, especially when compared to more severe injuries to the brain.

With this in mind, I would like to discard the concept of physical and structural injuries to the spine, jaw, and brain as the model for whiplash-based injury. Instead, I would like to explore the concept of the whiplash experience as a model of traumatization, with long-standing and at times permanent neurophysiological and neurochemical changes in the brain that are experience-based, rather than injury-based. In this model, these changes are triggered by a cascade of neural impulses and neurotransmitters precipitated by a continuous state of intense arousal, alternating with recurrence of the freeze response, resulting in turn from an unresolved perceived life threat in a state of relative helplessness. This is a dramatic departure from the long-standing and traditional concept of whiplash as spinal injury. It presents, however, a compelling and logical theory, bringing together the diverse elements of the whiplash syndrome into a cohesive whole.

Chapter 4

The Whiplash Syndrome II:
A Model for Traumatization

> I dreamed last night that I was playing basketball with a pro team, and all of the players had knives strapped to their arms and legs. Pretty soon we were all cut up, and there was blood all over everyone, and all over the floor. The ball was so slippery that it kept slipping out of everyone's hands.

This was a dream related to me by a patient who had awakened in a state of complete awareness while strapped down, intubated, and paralyzed shortly after induction of anesthesia, and who remained in this state of existential helplessness throughout a ninety-minute surgical procedure. Her symptoms consisted of all of the symptoms of the whiplash syndrome described in the previous chapter, including myofascial pain, bruxing, visual impairment, vertigo, cognitive impairment, and of course, post-traumatic stress disorder.

* * *

MEMORY MECHANISMS IN TRAUMA

Memory mechanisms play a critical role in forming the complex neurophysiological fabric of traumatization. The odds of a lasting memory being implanted in those centers of the brain related to memory storage is directly proportional to the arousal or emotional content of the experience that accompanied the event to be remembered.[1] One usually tends to remember important life events with little difficulty. Not only are they associated with specific meanings to us, but they are also usually associated with strong emotions, both negative and positive. Those in my generation tend to remember with vivid clarity what they were doing at the exact moment they learned that President Kennedy had been shot. We usually remember with remarkable detail the events of our weddings, the funerals of loved ones, the greatest moments of our children's success, the news that we have a critical illness, or the vivid experience of a serious physical injury. All of these events are associated with heightened emotions, alertness, or arousal. Animal experiments reveal that they learn certain tasks more quickly if the task is paired with an arousing stimulus instead of a neutral stimulus.

I would like to review arousal/memory mechanisms in the face of threat as presented in Chapter 2. As you will recall, the area of the brain most responsible for processing of memory associated with emotion is the amygdala, the small bulb-shaped nucleus at the anterior tip of the limbic system in the medial temporal lobe (see Figure 2.1). The primary role of the amygdala is the processing of sensory input from the body with regard to the arousal or emotional content of that information. Much of the information comes from the locus ceruleus, which has rich connections with the primary sensory organs of the head and proprioceptive receptors in the neck. Positioning of the head both in the act of orienting to sources of food, as well as sources of threat, is critical to accessing environmental sensory information via the organs of smell, taste, vision, hearing, and vestibular sensation. With sensory input via these sources, the amygdala evaluates the emotional meaning of the incoming information, and integrates the memory image of the event with the emotional experience.[2] The hippocampus, the center for verbal and conscious memory, forms a cognitive matrix for that memory image. The right orbitofrontal cortex then mediates the process of routing messages to appropriate areas of the cerebral cortex for more complex memory organization, and to brainstem and motor centers for organization of defensive behavioral patterns that ultimately, will assure survival.[3] If this response is successful, these patterns of motor behavior will be stored for use in future threatening experiences in brainstem centers that retain unconscious motor and conditioned procedural memories.

Declarative versus Nondeclarative Memory

Two clearly distinguishable and separate memory systems in the brain have been defined. Declarative or explicit memory is concerned with verbal and semantic memory for facts, events, and information—i.e., "knowing that."[4] It is conscious, intentional, and is the part that we use in acquiring information and a formal education. It contains subsystems for episodic memory related to personal experience, and semantic memory transmitted from another's experience, as in education. Damage to the hippocampus, the brain region probably most important in declarative memory, results in the inability to store new conscious information, as well as excessive responsiveness to environmental stimuli.[5,6] Posttraumatic amnesia is characterized by the loss of a segment of declarative memory. It is often one of the earliest functions lost in Alzheimer's disease and other organic dementias. Declarative memory is also affected and sometimes distorted by the emotional content of the associated experience, and may be notoriously inaccurate. This is clearly illustrated by the varying stories told by survivors of the same traumatic natural disaster or life event, and by the occasional change and distortion of old memories through new life experiences. Declarative memory probably represents only a small fraction of stored memory.

Nondeclarative, or implicit memory, is responsible for storing acquired skills, conditioned responses, and emotional associations—i.e., "knowing how." [4,7] It is unconscious, and governs much of that part of our daily activity that is automatic and instinctual, based on past experiences and training. The part of nondeclarative memory that serves skills and habits as well as conditioned sensorimotor responses is called procedural memory. All of the motor skills that we learn and never forget, such as musical, artistic, and athletic talents are stored in procedural memory. Procedural memories are readily acquired without intention, and retained forever without awareness, especially if they are linked to a coincident emotional event.[2] They are acquired and stored without the necessary involvement of conscious memory centers serving declarative memory, such as the hippocampus and prefrontal cortex. Motor skill memories are probably in part stored in the brainstem, cerebellum, and extrapyramidal centers controlling basic primitive postural reflexes.

Another type of nondeclarative memory is involved in the process of unconscious conditioned behavior. Conditioned responses or memories may involve the sensorimotor or autonomic nervous systems and are by definition unconscious. In Pavlov's classic experiment, the induction of consistent salivation in a dog by ringing a bell after pairing the bell with feeding is linked to nondeclarative memory mechanisms. Conditioned responses of this type require reinforcement by continued pairing of the external stimuli to maintain the conditioned behavior. If the bell rings enough times without presentation of the food, the salivation response will undergo extinction and will disappear. This type of conditioning, unlike most procedural memory, is not permanent. If, however, the paired stimuli include a component involving high arousal or emotion, it will take fewer trials of exposure to produce the conditioned behavior, and more trials of unpaired stimuli to extinguish it. In fact, if one of the stimuli represents a life-threatening event, the conditioned response may appear after one trial and never be extinguished. Conditioned responses are therefore clearly critical to the unconscious survival-based behavior of the organism. The conditioned response to acute trauma is specifically related to the events and symptom complex accompanying the whiplash syndrome. With these concepts of procedural and conditioned memory linked to arousal we can begin to reexamine the whiplash syndrome in an entirely new light.

SOMATIC RESPONSES TO STRESS

At or even before the moment of impact of two automobiles, the occupants undergo a predictable series of neurophysiological events. Whether or not the impact was anticipated based on the presence of preceding sensory input may have a bearing on these events and the resulting symptoms. Attempts to determine whether symptoms are worse in the presence or absence of a warning have had mixed results. The prevailing opinion is that anticipation allowing the ability of the person to brace for the impact should diminish injuries. At least one study suggests that the element of surprise resulted in more severe injuries.[8] Symptoms indeed may differ in these two situations, but the outcomes are probably similar. Sensory input usually involves visual or auditory awareness of the impending crash and may have an effect on the content of subsequent memories related to the trauma. In either case, within milliseconds, the thalamus receives a barrage of messages from visual, auditory, proprioceptive, and vestibular sensory organs, which are then sent to the amygdala for analysis of emotional content. Based on the potentially life-threatening nature of the event, and with input from locus ceruleus, the systemic release of epinephrine from adrenal medulla along with brainstem norepinephrine will trigger the physiological sequence of the fight/flight response, within both the central nervous system and somatic end organs.

The systemic manifestations of the fight/flight response are of course predictable, but worth reviewing in the context of the accident itself. The eyes will widen, the pupils will dilate, and the eyes diverge slightly in order to achieve maximal visual access to the threat. The pulse, systolic blood pressure, and cardiac output will markedly increase. Skeletal muscles will exhibit increased tone in preparation for action, but at the same time will be subjected to powerful forces involving stretch and torque in a variety of directions. As the car is moved in one direction as a result of the impact, inertia will inhibit the body from immediately moving, resulting in an apparent movement in the direction of the impact. Stretch receptors in muscles on the side *opposite* the source of impact will be activated, resulting in selective intense contraction of these muscles on a reflex basis through the gamma motoneuron circuitry. As the rate of acceleration decreases, the body will then rebound, moving next in the direction of the impact, and activating stretch receptors on the side of the impact, but to a lesser degree. Based on any rotational positions of the body at the moment of impact, torque forces will also activate varied muscle groups on both sides of the body, causing a complex and diffuse pattern of muscle bracing that is predictably asymmetrical and regional in distribution. The rapid acceleration/deceleration forces in varied directions will cause marked perturbation of vestibular receptors in the semicircular canals. Activation of vestibulospinal pathways will further contribute to postural muscle bracing patterns based on directions of movement of the head. Proprioceptive input from ligaments, tendons, and muscles will result in further reflex postural holding patterns. Those parts of the body involved in the control of the vehicle, especially the hands on the steering wheel and feet on brake or accelerator pedals, will react based on procedural memory patterns of motor driving behavior. The resulting motor response will involve bracing, clenching, or turning of the body in reflex reaction to visual, vestibular, and proprioceptive input from sense organs in the head, neck, and muscles of the body.

At the same time, the marked shift in sympathetic tone will inhibit the vegetative functions of the viscera and cardiovascular system. With the MVA victim in an acute state of fight/flight readiness, and subjected to powerful gravitational forces, the next physiological de-

mand calls for completion of the high level physical activity required
to dissipate the effect of adrenergic arousal on the body. At this point
the meaning of the event and the relative empowerment of the victim
to pursue the physical activity of the fight/flight response become
critical. The basic concept of transport in a vehicle of conveyance actually becomes a profoundly important issue.

THE MEANING OF SPEED

Vehicular Transport and Society

Although human beings have traveled in wheeled vehicles drawn
by horses or other animals for centuries, the speed of travel has been
generally slow, and the distances short. The advent of mechanized,
relatively high-speed travel with the invention of the steam engine in
the nineteenth century has had a remarkable effect on human society.
Distances have shrunk, the pace of life and the amount "accom-
plished" in a unit of time have increased, and humans have become
accustomed to the unnerving sensations of traveling at a high rate of
speed. Nevertheless, a person's first experience with the sensations
of rapid acceleration and centrifugal force is often arousing and even
frightening. Fear of flying in an airplane for the first time is common,
and even repeated exposure with benign experiences does not always
extinguish the fear. Amusement park rides are often terrifying before
they become exhilarating. Nothing in our physiological evolution
prepares us for this particular experience of acute and violent vestibular stimulation. Although the peculiar syndrome involving pain with
emotional and cognitive symptoms associated with vehicular accidents has probably been around since the Roman chariots, the first
apparent recorded reference to this condition probably relates to
"Railroad Spine," referred to in Chapter 3.[9] During that period of the
nineteenth century, this condition was believed to fall into the nebu-
lous category of the neuroses, and as with present day whiplash, was
predominantly seen in women.

As mechanized transport has transformed the twentieth-century
world, vehicles have assumed roles and meanings far more varied
and complex than simply a means of travel. This is especially true in
the case of the automobile, which in its century of evolution has progressed from a curiosity to a sign of power and control, a symbol of

wealth and accomplishment, and a source of thrill and exhilaration. In much of the civilized world, the automobile and its operation is considered a God-given right, and a necessity of life. On the other hand, those individuals subjected to the forces associated with rapid mechanized transport that suddenly operate outside of the boundaries of control seldom consider the experience exhilarating. They tend to report the experience of panic or arousal in situations involving loss of control of a motor vehicle, when the crash is averted. If a crash does occur, however, they frequently undergo an experience of numbing or shock for a period of time. As first reported in cases of "Railroad Spine," the effects of sudden high speed and unexpected changes in velocity or direction may produce distressing and long-standing symptoms in certain individuals, especially if this loss of control culminates in a crash.

The increasing frequency of soft tissue injuries in MVAs, the relative resistance to treatment of victims of whiplash, and the incredible costs of their medical care suggests that some unique process is taking place when the human body is subjected to these forces in the context of mechanized transport. Yet a paradox exists in cases of loss of control of a motor vehicle, even associated with a crash, when the operation of the vehicle is connected with an environment of aggression, competition, or intentional risk-taking, or when the driver is inebriated at the time of the crash. Although meaningful statistics are not available, there seems to be no significant incidence of true whiplash syndrome in race car or stunt drivers involved in impact crashes, despite the occurrence of significant physical injuries, cerebral concussions, and life-threatening situations. In the well over 5,000 cases of whiplash that I have treated, I have never seen manifestations of the whiplash syndrome in a person substantially under the influence of alcohol at the time of the accident. The common denominator in cases of MVAs in which whiplash syndrome develops, therefore, appears to be the occurrence of the accident when the individual is in a state of helplessness.

The Automobile As a Threat

Most automobile drivers, fortunately, respect the risks associated with the operation of their car, and realize that bodily injury and death occur with distressing frequency with their use. Admittedly, this appropriate sense of vulnerability seems to be uniquely lacking during the teen years, but it seems to develop in most people with the acquisition of what we define as maturity. Although automobile manufacturers have made admirable progress in improving the handling of cars, there is always a fine line in their control that, if crossed, results in the immediate condition of complete helplessness. Most drivers have experienced this sensation of loss of control at some point in their driving careers, and having done so, will never again feel the complete sense of driver confidence that they did before that experience. Even a small collision will usually be enough to change forever the driver's sense of safety in a car. Obviously gender, personality, and past life experiences have a major effect on the evolution of this sense of awareness of vulnerability in a car. Nevertheless, for most drivers, operation of a car takes place with a variable sense of risk and helplessness.

In the context of the fight/flight/freeze response, a state of helplessness by definition eliminates the option of fighting or fleeing, and obviously neither of these two options exists when one automobile is impacted by another. The event itself, however, is intrinsically life threatening, and will inevitably trigger the appropriate physiological responses of the fight/flight response. In a state of helplessness, the initiation of the fight/flight physiological events will just as inevitably trigger the freeze response, which I feel occurs in a substantial number of MVA victims.

Detailed histories of the initial subjective experiences of MVA victims often reflect the frequency of symptoms of freezing. The immediate experiences of the whiplash victim during the period surrounding the impact of the automobiles are often remembered in vague and even surreal terms. During the moments after the impact, many patients will describe a sense of shock, confusion, and detachment, often with no describable emotional tone. "Numbness" is the word most often used to describe the quality of this experience. On rare occasions, the patient will describe the sensation of being "full of adrenaline," or "shaking all over," but an immediate feeling of arousal is uncommon. Often the memory for specific events is vague and unclear, and details of the impact are often remembered piecemeal or out of sequence.

Occasionally a sense of detached calm is present, and the victims may appear remarkably rational and in control of themselves. More often, however, victims will describe a feeling of helplessness and of being overwhelmed. Others will have a sense of unreality, saying to themselves, "How could this happen to me?" On occasion, a number of my patients have described frank "out-of-body" experiences. Witnesses may describe victims as dazed. Attempts by the accident victim to describe the events of the MVA at a later time will frequently reflect the fragmented nature of their recall. Many of these experiences fall into the category of derealization or depersonalization, symptoms typical of dissociation (see Chapter 8).

THE PHYSIOLOGY OF TRAUMATIZATION

How then does traumatization occurring in the context of an MVA explain the varied and multisystemic symptom complex of the whiplash syndrome? The experience of trauma primarily involves arousal and memory mechanisms as outlined earlier. Aberrations of memory in trauma involve both declarative and nondeclarative memory, and are characterized by both exaggerated and impaired memory functions.[2] In many instances, victims of trauma are amnestic for various events associated with the traumatic event.[2] Memory of the event itself is frequently distorted and inaccurate. Many adults abused as children have no specific memory of the trauma itself, and have a vague sense only of being traumatized. When memories themselves are "recovered," they often are remarkably distorted. This distortion or suppression of traumatic memories may be proportional to the severity of the freeze response, or dissociation at the time of the trauma. Enhancement of memories of the event may also be prominent, leading to involuntary resurfacing of these memories in a variety of settings. Arousal linked to the conscious memories of sensory experiences of the trauma leads to the laying down of a powerful feedback circuit within associated brain centers, in part probably involving locus ceruleus, amygdala, and hypothalamus.[1] This may result in the triggering of recurrent and intrusive memories of the trauma with even nonspecific arousal, and the triggering of arousal by even nonspecific events or perceptions reminiscent of the trauma.

This arousal/memory link in trauma also may be enhanced by nondeclarative and declarative memories of past trauma with links to the immediate event, such as prior experience with MVAs. Specific procedural memories of sensorimotor experiences arising from both current and past related trauma may also be incorporated into this newly activated circuitry. Subsequent arousal may then trigger recurrence of these experiential memories, such as pain, dizziness, and the protective neuromuscular bracing response associated with the MVA. These experiences and sensations may then be incorporated in the arousal/memory circuitry.

Kindling and Trauma

The mechanism by which this self-sustaining feedback circuit is established may well be related to the physiological phenomenon of kindling. The term kindling was developed from the description of spontaneous combustion of materials reaching a certain critical temperature. The physiological model was developed in rats by applying a repetitive electrical stimulus to an area of the brain with specific frequency and intensity.[10] Although each stimulus was insufficient to trigger a convulsion, if the stimuli were applied with a critical frequency, they would summate and trigger a seizure. In addition, if kindled seizures were induced in newborn rats with many repetitions, the rats would exhibit the tendency for spontaneous seizures that thereafter would be self-perpetuating, and would occur without any stimulus. In other words, these rats developed a relatively permanent change in the excitability of neuronal networks within the kindled part of their brain. The brain region most susceptible to kindling is the amygdala.

In the case of PTSD, the repetitive neural input to the feedback loop associated with recurrent memory events may well derive from the sustained high-level adrenergic arousal persisting as a result of the undischarged freeze response, and the resulting uninhibited autonomic cycling between hyperarousal and freeze/dissociation. Threat-related information generated both by internal memory and external experiential cues would routinely activate the amygdala that in turn would interpret the resulting emotion-based memories as threatening, resulting in the triggering of arousal once again. The result would be the spectrum of memory events seen in PTSD: flashbacks, intrusive memories, cue-related memories, and nightmares. Another result would be the arousal symptoms of PTSD: anxiety, panic attacks, phobias of events and places reminiscent of the trauma, memory and situation-induced arousal, mood changes, irritability, stimulus sensitivity, exaggerated startle, and insomnia. In individuals with significant prior unresolved traumatic stress experiences, modulation of the organized response to threat may be diminished due to impaired development of the right orbitofrontal cortex, leading to impaired regulation of arousal/memory mechanisms. Under these circumstances, establishment of kindled connections between centers of arousal (locus ceruleus, amygdala) and memory (hippocampus, sensorimotor centers for procedural memory) may be established (see Figure 4.1), leading to increasing potentiation of these pathways by internal as well as external cues, and worsening of clinical symptoms.

The frequent delay in onset of symptoms of PTSD after a traumatic event is quite consistent with the concept of kindling as an evolving neurophysiological process. Similarly, the tendency for PTSD to change in both the nature of the predominant symptoms and the occasional worsening of the condition is consistent with kindling, a process that by definition changes neural excitability and eventually becomes self-sustaining without further external input. Delay in onset, change in basic characteristics, and the spontaneous worsening of memory and arousal-related symptoms are all typical of the progress of PTSD symptoms in the whiplash syndrome. The same characteristics are also typical of the cognitive and somatic symptoms of whiplash, which often do not appear for a variable period after the MVA, and may evolve and change character over many months. Other authors have also addressed the concept of kindling in relationship to the physiological basis for the development of PTSD.[11,12,13]

Cognitive Deficits in Trauma

The DSM-IV criteria for the diagnosis of PTSD do not adequately take into account the complex interaction of emotional and somatic experiences in an MVA. Blanchard and Hickling have advocated use of the designation of a subsyndromal form of PTSD in MVA victims.[14] Their criteria for this subsyndromal form specify inclusion of criteria for Section B (reexperiencing), and either C (avoidance), or D (hyperarousal), to establish the diagnosis. Even acknowledgment of a subsyndromal form of PTSD may not fully recognize the fact that a remarkably prolonged freeze response, or period of posttraumatic dissociation, may mask many of the symptoms of arousal and reexperiencing for an indeterminate period of time, thereby preventing the criteria-based diagnosis of PTSD. Under these circumstances, the predominant

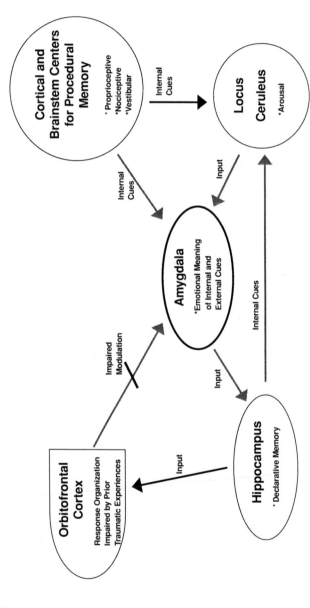

FIGURE 4.1. Theoretical model of arousal/memory kindling in post-traumatic stress disorder. Imprinting of declarative and procedural memories for the traumatic event by lack of completion of the freeze discharge leads to perpetuation of a kindled neuronal loop incorporating locus ceruleus, amygdala, hippocampus and brainstem, and cortical centers for procedural memory. Internal memory cues, both declarative and procedural, serve to potentiate arousal. The impairment of the modulating influence of a poorly developed right orbitofrontal cortex due to prior life trauma may potentiate this process.

symptoms may be those of numbing, distraction, and cognitive symptoms usually attributed to a concussion or minor traumatic brain injury (see Chapter 3). Even in the absence of any conceivable head trauma, PTSD has been associated with substantial cognitive deficits of a severity and similarity sufficient to make the diagnosis of a head injury on neuropsychological test batteries.[15,16] Cognitive deficits attributable only to PTSD in the face of documented traumatic events have been demonstrated in such occurrences as terrorist attacks, imprisonment, vehicular accidents, and combat-related sinking of ships.[17,18,19] These cognitive deficits have a solid theoretical base in the neurohumoral changes triggered by trauma. Trauma has been shown to interfere with declarative memory, but not nondeclarative or procedural memory.[1] This phenomenon appears to be related to the input of norepinephrine to the amygdala, allowing the brain to differentiate the emotional meaning of the incoming information. High activity within the amygdala inhibits storage and synthesis of declarative memory within the hippocampus while facilitating storage of memory linked to the norepinephrine-induced arousal.[3] In addition, the release of high levels of endorphins in the brain as part of the response to this arousal further interferes with memory consolidation.[20] The result is a state of impaired declarative memory storage in the face of enhanced storage of trauma-related memory, most of it nondeclarative. In addition, high levels of cortisol have a direct inhibitory, and in fact neurotoxic effect on hippocampal structures, thereby enhancing the inhibitory effect on declarative memory.[21,22,23] The result is the exaggeration of trauma-related memories that, in fact, become intrusive at the expense of conscious declarative memory processes, and contribute to the documented memory deficits in PTSD.[15]

As noted, endogenous opioids may also be involved in memory dysfunction in PTSD. Stress-induced analgesia is a well-known accompaniment of severe trauma. Soldiers with severe wounds have been noted to deny the need for morphine for some time after their injuries.[24] This is consistent with previously mentioned studies that show that both norepinephrine and endorphins are released after exposure to severe stress. Animal studies reveal that animals unable to escape a threatening situation and which exhibit withdrawal/despair—i.e., the freeze response—suffer from significant impairment of memory.[20] In these animals, both the freeze response and panic interfered with memory processing, suggesting that both epinephrine and endorphins contribute to this deficit. Van der Kolk has postulated that the freeze/numbing response in animals exposed to prolonged severe and inescapable stress may be analogous to dissociation in humans exposed to trauma, and that dissociation may also be mediated by endogenous opiates.[2] Excessive endorphin release may, therefore, play a role in the well-documented deficits in memory noted in patients suffering from PTSD. Traumatic memory intrusion may also contribute to the documented deficits in attention, concentration, and multitask thinking in PTSD. In addition, arousal triggered by recurrent and kindled traumatic memories induces release of norepinephrine that once again activates the memory/arousal feedback circuit as well as the hypothalamic/pituitary/adrenal axis (HPA), and sustains the cognitive deficits of PTSD. These concepts challenge the assumption in the whiplash syndrome that specific and documented cognitive dysfunction is by definition indicative of traumatic brain injury, especially in low velocity accidents.

Trauma and the Postconcussion Syndrome

Another matter of concern in the concept of concussion is the varied symptom complex commonly referred to as the postconcussion syndrome. This is a vague group of complaints that typically includes atypical headache, visual complaints usually involving blurring of vision, balance disturbance, tinnitus, dizziness and vertigo, orthostatic lightheadedness, and mood disturbances. These mood changes have been recognized to contain many of the symptoms of PTSD, and include irritability, stimulus sensitivity to noise and lights, sleep disturbance, fatigue, and depression. Researchers have begun to recognize this association between PTSD and the elements of the postconcussion syndrome.[18,25] In MVA-related concussion, all of the symptoms associated with postconcussion syndrome can be explained by the concept of traumatization. In this model, the end organs involved in receiving the necessary information for reflex self-protective behavior in an MVA are primarily those sensory centers of the head and neck. These sources of sensory input include the extraocular muscles of the eyes, the vestibular apparatus of the inner ear and brainstem, the hearing apparatus of the inner ear, the autonomic nervous system and its control of peripheral blood vessels, and the muscles of the head, neck, and shoulder girdle. The sense of smell may also record olfactory information for further reference for survival. Sensory input from these end organs at the time of a whiplash will be incorporated in the arousal response and then in the kindled circuitry involving arousal and procedural memory for the event.

Binocular Dysfunction

As we have noted, under the influence of peripheral epinephrine and brainstem norepinephrine, the eyes will diverge at the moment of trauma or immediate threat, and the pupils of the eyes will dilate. This takes place by reflex activation of the extraocular muscles and the circular muscles that make up the iris of the eye. This response is as automatic as the stretch reflex, and serves to maximize the field of vision in the situation of threat or danger. This ocular reflex inevitably accompanies any arousal threat, including that of an MVA. As with other events associated with arousal, it is frozen in the event of the freeze response, and dissipated by its physiological discharge in the event of survival after freezing.

Applying the concept that retention of traumatic arousal occurs because of impaired freeze discharge, the ocular and pupillary changes triggered by traumatic arousal will continue to be linked in the evolving feedback circuit between centers of arousal and those for procedural memory, the storehouse for motor skills and habits. Under these conditions, any arousal, whether linked to the other memories of the accident or even occurring in the stresses of everyday life, will nonspecifically trigger ocular divergence and pupillary dilatation. In fact, these are basically the clinical findings that have been documented in examinations of patients with postconcussion vision abnormalities (see Chapter 3). Such patients almost inevitably are found to have impaired binocular movements and convergence insufficiency representing the persistence of variable tonic ocular divergence. In this model, however, these changes are not the result of brain injury per se, but rather the incorporation of the eye muscles in the neuromuscular/arousal/memory conditioned and kindled circuit of unresolved trauma.

Vestibular and Autonomic Dysfunction

The same theory applies to all of the remaining manifestations of the whiplash syndrome. Because of the intense forces of acceleration and deceleration in an MVA, the vestibular and proprioceptive sensory apparatus of the inner ears and musculoskeletal system are subjected to massive sensory input. Once again, linking of arousal and memory to the conditioned activation of the vestibular system results in the appearance of vertigo, dizziness, and balance disturbance under conditions of arousal. In addition, any quick movement of the head results in vestibular input.

Since the particular and unique vestibular input at the time of the MVA is stored in procedural memory linked to arousal, movements of the head that coincidentally access the MVA-related movement pattern will trigger arousal and evoke the sensation of vertigo and loss of balance. So-called "cervical vertigo" may therefore arise from muscles of the neck involved originally in bracing patterns of the accident. Activation of bracing and movement patterns involving these muscles may arouse procedural memories of the vestibular stimulation experienced in the accident and linked at that moment to perceived life threat, thereby repeatedly inducing vertigo with head movement. Vertigo in this model therefore represents survival-based procedural memory. This phenomenon may explain the absence of objective findings in many cases of positional vertigo in MVAs.

A labile and unstable autonomic nervous system is known to accompany PTSD. The primary measures in chronic cases involve documentation of unstable pulse and blood pressure responses to nonspecific arousal stimuli, sounds, pictures, or even smells reminiscent of the trauma, or even guided imagery of the trauma. Electrodermal skin response has also been used with some success in identifying PTSD autonomic overresponders.[26]

Victims of PTSD are known to cycle in and out of arousal and dissociation, the former associated with adrenergic dominance, the latter with endorphinergic and probably selective vagal influences. In the early stages after an MVA, an exaggerated sympathetic response may be at its most dramatic. I have documented many patients with systolic blood pressures over 170 mmHg with no history of hypertension, and with pulses of 120 to 140 bpm at rest. Most of these patients have been in acute arousal and anxiety, with many symptoms of the arousal portion of PTSD. On the other hand, those patients presenting with characteristic of sustained freeze and dissociation will generally present with low systolic blood pressure, occasional bradycardia, and frequent orthostatic hypotension and dizziness. Actual syncope is not uncommon in these individuals. Many of these dissociated patients will suffer from dramatic alternating constipation and diarrhea, and occasionally from symptoms of peptic acid disease.

Autonomic instability, I believe, is a secondary, conditioned phenomenon linked to the arousal/ memory feedback circuit of traumatization, with the numbing and the dissociation of the freeze response often associated with cholinergic symptoms. The basis for this is found in the role of selected brainstem vagal centers, and is discussed in more detail in Chapter 8.

Neuromuscular Dysfunction and Myofascial Pain

The other end organ system involved in traumatization in the whiplash syndrome, one that is totally ignored in consideration of MVA-related PTSD, is the neuromuscular system. Posttraumatic headache, and cervical and lumbosacral spinal pain constitute the primary symptoms related to whiplash. This pain has been attributed to injuries to muscles, tendons, ligaments, intervertebral discs, spinal facet joints, and nerve roots.[27] In the final analysis, however, the prolonged and intractable pain of whiplash I feel is eventually attributable primarily to the condition of myofascial pain. The relationship of myofascial pain in the whiplash syndrome to the arousal/memory link in trauma is quite analogous to the involvement of other end organ systems with procedural memory for the traumatic event. At the instant of impact, selected muscles are stretched in a coordinated and synchronous pattern depending specifically on the direction of the initial acceleration of the body. Input from the stretched muscle spindle initiates contraction of alpha muscle fibers through stimulation of the gamma motoneuron system at the level of the spinal cord. At the instant of this selective grouped alpha muscle activation, proprioceptive input from the associated musculotendinous units travels to the cerebellum via group I and/or group II afferent fibers. In response to this sensory information related to changes in velocity, cerebellar nuclei then provide neuronal input to the thalamus, brainstem vestibular nuclei, and basal ganglia. These centers in turn provide reflex regulation of complex postural changes via the spinal cord anterior horn cells and gamma motoneuron system.

In addition, input from the thalamus to the amygdala facilitates assessment of the emotional content of the experience. Since the sudden velocity changes accompanying the MVA carry the implication of imminent life threat, arousal via brainstem norepinephrine pathways will accompany thalamic input to the amygdala, setting up the scenario of the full-blown fight/flight response. If physiological freezing accompanies the completion of the MVA, as it often does, the experience of the complex neuromuscular response to the velocity forces of the accident will be incorporated into procedural memory in its exact form, just as will any learned motor skill. In addition, these patterned neuromuscular responses will be reinforced by their association with high arousal, and therefore will be relatively permanent.[28] Finally, these self-protective movement patterns will be incorporated into the kindled arousal/memory circuitry of traumatization.

Thereafter, memories of the accident, familiar stimuli reminiscent of the accident, dreams of the accident, arousal related to those memories, and eventually nonspecific arousal will tend to facilitate procedural neuromuscular memory of regional protective muscular bracing patterns from the MVA. Reflex activation of muscle groups will then be produced in a pattern mimicking that associated with the body movements caused by the accident. The MVA victim will experience involuntary tightening of a selective group of regional muscles in a repetitive pattern, triggered by arousal, dreams, driving activities, or memories of the accident. Repetitive use of those muscles in any other activities may trigger arousal and reciprocal reflex muscle spasm as the sensorimotor arm of the kindled circuit is activated. This phenomenon explains the occasional triggering of remote traumatic memories by massage or other types of body therapy. Since muscles are designed to contract briefly on a reciprocal basis with their opponents, involuntary sustained contraction of muscle groups on the basis of arousal-generated reflex input from postural centers of the brain sets up a condition of energy failure. This leads to an accumulation of metabolic waste products in muscle fibers, release of kinins and other chemical pain generators, and a condition of relative ischemia in the involved fibers. The result is regional myofascial pain perpetuated by the same kindled feedback circuitry producing the symptoms of PTSD.

Cephalic Myofascial Pain

In any MVA, the muscles of the head, neck, and jaw are invariably the most involved in residual long-term regional myofascial pain. Whether the mechanism of the accident involves a rear-end, head-on, or rollover impact, neck pain, headache, and jaw pain usually are inevitable. In the velocity-change model of physical injury to these structures, the cause is felt to lie in the pendular effect of the skull on the neck, rendering these structures more vulnerable to damaging forces. This does not, however, explain the same phenomenon in low velocity accidents, or when the head and neck were not subjected to unusual forces based on the particular dynamics of the accident.

Another explanation lies in the intimate neural association of the locus ceruleus with sensory end organs and especially joint proprioceptors of the head and cervical spine. These sensory receptors provide the locus ceruleus with information about environmental threat through positional orientation of the head and its sensory apparatus. The orienting reflex, a gradual side-to-side rotation of the head allowing scanning of the environment for information utilizing all of the sense organs of the head, is a basic and universal instinctual motor pattern in all species. Muscles of the head and neck are therefore intimately involved in sensory information access in all situations, both with regard to feeding and to fight/flight survival.

Activation of cephalic and cervical muscles with associated bracing in response to threat renders them uniquely vulnerable to the conditioned inclusion of this bracing pattern in the arousal feedback circuit, with subsequent persistent cervical myofascial pain. Jaw clenching is a primitive arousal reflex, with its roots lying deeply in instinctual patterns involving use of the teeth and jaw in alimentation, and as both offensive and defensive weapons in animals. The muscles of mastication in addition are embryologically derived from branchial arch muscles, and originally were involved in the process of respiration. Unconscious bruxing after an MVA therefore is incorporated into the nonspecific protective muscular bracing patterns linked to unresolved arousal, leading to the well-known but perplexing condition of TMJ syndrome. This bruxing occurs mainly during sleep, a period of time where the day's experiences are integrated with old declarative and procedural memories for the purpose of perpetuating survival-directed behavior.

CONCLUSION

Clinical experience suggests that many victims involved in MVAs experience dissociation, or freezing, at the moment of the accident. Dissociation is known to be a major predictor of eventual development of PTSD, and is felt to be the equivalent of the freeze response seen in animals. For reasons as yet unclear, the human species, unlike creatures in the wild, tends not to go through the stereotyped and instinctual neuromuscular discharge of the autonomic arousal of the freeze response in the face of trauma.

The physiological model of kindling presents a compelling rationale for the symptom complex of PTSD. Stored autonomic energy from a truncated freeze response might well provide the impetus and fuel for development of kindling in trauma. The experimental model of kindling, of course, entails the application of an external stimulus to trigger development of the resulting self-perpetuating circuitry. In this case, the external stimulus is experientially related to sensory input rather than to external application of an electrical impulse. Involvement of arousal and procedural memory circuitry is clearly implicated in the model of traumatic kindling. Linking of these arousal and memory centers with those of the sensory end organs involved in the traumatic experience will predictably result in a cyclical and kindled repetition of somatic symptoms representative of the intense sensory input experienced at the moment of trauma. The entire process represents an abortive attempt by primitive brain centers to integrate events of the traumatic experience into memory for the purpose of survival.

This process provides a unitary hypothesis for the myriad symptoms of whiplash. It also provides a model for the concept of somatization, one of the more prominent comorbid conditions seen in PTSD. In this model, myofascial pain is caused by arousal-activated descending motor input from reflex motor centers of the brainstem to the spinal anterior horn cell, linked to sustained arousal associated with unresolved discharge of the freeze response. The specific distribution of the involved muscles is based on anatomical and physiological procedural memory patterns of the neuromuscular defensive bracing response to movement patterns of the MVA. Those muscle groups activated by the stretch reflex to contract in response to the velocity changes in the accident will continue to brace in the face of arousal or memory input related to the trauma. As a phenomenon of central rather than peripheral origin, this hypothesis explains the remarkable lack of consistency or specificity of findings with investigation of the peripheral portion of the motor unit in myofascial pain using electrophysiological, chemical, and biopsy studies. It also explains the frequent regional persistence of myofascial pain, and its variable lack of response to peripheral forms of treatment, which typically provides only temporary benefit.

Similarly, vestibular, auditory, visual, and autonomic symptoms of the postconcussion syndrome may represent somatic experiences of the MVA that are stored in procedural memory and linked to arousal circuitry. These symptoms will be perpetuated by any head movement reminiscent of the trauma, and also by nonspecific arousal or by declarative memory of the accident. Although focal brain or end organ injury certainly may contribute to some of these symptoms, their frequently delayed onset and occurrence in low velocity accidents supports their etiology in the neurophysiology of traumatization.

Although minor traumatic brain injury may be a cause of specific and sometimes persisting cognitive deficits in victims of MVAs, cognitive impairment in the whiplash syndrome is also explainable by the mechanisms of dissociation, attention deficit, and thought intrusion seen in PTSD. In very low velocity accidents, these physiological events associated with trauma are more than likely the primary etiology for significant cognitive symptoms and impairment.

Chapter 5

Trauma and Brain Plasticity

Sandy had been injured in a rollover accident and had suffered from a long period of cognitive impairment, driving phobias, sleep disturbance, and headaches. She had received several years of treatment, both cognitive therapy for her minor traumatic brain injury, and somatically based trauma therapy, including Eye Movement Desensitization and Reprocessing (EMDR) and Somatic Experiencing (SE). Although she continued to experience problems with memory and speed of information processing, she had managed to complete a master's level degree during her recovery, and went on to train as a skilled SE practitioner. Her phobic and arousal symptoms had largely cleared, except for difficulties with sleep maintenance. Two years after the accident, she lost control of her car on an icy road, and ran head-on into a tree. She totally destroyed her car, and suffered multiple bruises. At the scene she immediately applied her therapeutic skills, and effectively discharged the intense shock of the accident through a period of trembling and shaking.

A fellow therapist met her at the emergency room and continued to assist her in discharging the shock of the trauma. Although she experienced a predictable period of pain, anxiety, and fatigue, she never went through the prolonged and painful recovery that she had experienced after the first accident. One might speculate that her neurophysiological response to a severe traumatic event had been significantly and perhaps permanently altered by prior therapy designed to reduce vulnerability to fear conditioning.

* * *

The concept of trauma and its effects on the central nervous system and on human behavior has undergone dramatic and cyclical changes throughout the history of psychiatry. Theories of causation have fluctuated radically from psychological to physiological, from chemical brain alterations to impairment of willpower, from issues of secondary gain to malingering. The frequent shifts in bias and emphasis often have reflected the basic societal trends of the time. They have also been influenced by the culture or country represented by the most influential psychiatric theoreticians during that particular period of time. A fascinating and comprehensive review of the history of the concept of trauma in psychiatry may be found in van der Kolk, Weisaeth, and van der Hart.[1] A brief review of this history will serve as a background to the exciting and relatively recent reemergence of research into the neurophysiological bases for traumatization, and the development of the theory of post-traumatic stress disorder (PTSD) as a permanent change in brain physiology and structure.

THE HISTORY OF
POST-TRAUMATIC STRESS DISORDER
IN PSYCHIATRY

The fields of neurology and psychiatry evolved from a single discipline in the latter part of the nineteenth century, with the earlier clinicians in these specialties dealing with both physical diseases of the central nervous systems and diseases of the emotions or neuroses. Although theories of hysteria had emerged in prior decades, much of the important early work in this area took place in the Salpetriere Hospital in Paris. There the neuropsychiatrists Charcot and Janet first recognized that patients with hysteria appeared to have the basis for their symptoms in histories of childhood trauma.

Charcot first identified the association of hysteria with the phenomenon of dissociation, although he approached the concept from a purely neurological point of view, considering it a hereditary degenerative process.[2] Janet expanded the concepts of dissociation in trauma and postulated that intense emotional experience interfered with integration of memory into awareness.[3] He believed that these emotional experiences caused memories associated with them to be split off, or dissociated, from consciousness and to be stored instead as physical sensations of arousal and panic or as visual memories, such as flashbacks or nightmares. He also felt that subsequent efforts to keep these memories out of consciousness led to a gradual disintegration in personal functioning.[4] Thus, he introduced the roles of dissociation and memory into traumatization and addressed the potentially permanent and progressive nature of the disorder.

The Austrian neuropsychiatrist, Sigmund Freud, adopted many of these concepts from the Salpetriere in his early papers and initially acknowledged the association of conversion hysteria with childhood sexual abuse.[5] When he presented these findings and opinions to his Viennese colleagues, however, he was met with a storm of criticism, reflecting the cultural rigidity of his Victorian times and the unwillingness of the psychiatric community to acknowledge the pervasiveness of child abuse in existing middle-class society.[6]

As Freud developed his theory of psychoanalysis around the premise of repressed infantile sexuality, he progressively abandoned the concept of traumatization as a physiological disturbance of memory associated with dissociation. Instead, he related hysteria to active repression of the sexual and aggressive fantasies of the Oedipal complex with the mother, and denied the validity of reports of childhood sexual abuse in his hysterical patients.[7] The almost universal acceptance of psychoanalytic theory by the field of psychiatry resulted in the almost total rejection of the effect of child abuse and trauma on personality development, character traits, and psychiatric illness for almost eighty years.

Although the two world wars brought back to reality the fact that overwhelming life trauma resulted in profound emotional dysfunction, sporadic attempts to relate this association in a clinical setting were overwhelmed by the prevailing concepts of psychoanalytic theory. An exception was the work of Kardiner, a psychoanalyst who attempted to restructure his theories of war neurosis based on his observations of the pervasive hypervigilance and sensitivity to environmental stimuli of his patients. He actually introduced the concept of a *physioneurosis* related to trauma exposure, and commented on the progressive nature of the syndrome in many of his patients.[8] Kardiner documented many of the peculiar maladaptive traits of trauma victims that would later be incorporated into current definitions of PTSD. World War II afforded the opportunity to study traumatization in soldiers and concentration camp inmates. These studies in general documented the catastrophic effects of severe trauma on subsequent general health, and on the capacity to tolerate stress in later life.[9,10] Many of the postwar clinical investigators who studied these effects of trauma had themselves been part of wartime or concentration camp experiences.[1]

The Vietnam War resulted in another resurgence of interest in the effects of traumatic stress. This in turn rekindled interest in the work of Kardiner, and in 1980 led to an attempt to compile a list of symptoms related to trauma from the existing literature into a unitary syndrome. The new name for this syndrome was Post-traumatic Stress Disorder, and it was included for the first time in the *Diagnostic and Statistical Manual of Mental Disorders,* Third Edition (DSM-III). At the same time, attention was finally given to the previously ignored and relatively vast population of traumatized women and children.[11,12] Revisions of the definition of PTSD in the DSM (DSM-III-R, 1987, and DSM-IV, 1994) have continued to clarify and focus the epidemiology and clinical features of PTSD, but still have not completely defined the symptom of dissociation as specifically related to traumatic stress (see Chapter 6).

Since 1980, there has been an explosion of interest and research into the effects of trauma on the human brain and psyche, with the establishment of numerous journals and the publication of many books solely devoted to the study of human traumatic stress. Particularly noteworthy has been the increasing emphasis on the neurochemical, neurohumoral, and neurophysiological changes produced by the experience of trauma and the resulting breakdown of the separation of psychological and biological processes in mental illness. Physiological and behavioral studies in animals exposed to extreme stress have contributed greatly to the expanding knowledge of the basic science of trauma.[13] The movement of trauma research away from the psychoanalytic model has resulted in an increased awareness of the prevalence of trauma in all societies, and its pervasive effects on dysfunctional social and personal behavior. It has also fostered further research in the growing area of brain plasticity, not only in the face of physical damage from stroke or injury, but also associated with exposure to extreme stress.

THE DEVELOPING BRAIN

Plasticity of selected brain centers implies that sensory input specific to those centers influences their structure and can induce actual anatomical and neurochemical change. A large body of literature addresses the effect of sensory experience in animals on development or regression of brain structure, especially during the critical period of early brain development. Schore has assembled a vast portion of this research in both animals and humans, and has integrated it into a compelling theory of the effect of maternal-infant interaction on the structure and function of the developing brain.[14] Emphasizing neurophysiological aspects of development, Schore explores the effects of complex patterns of interaction between infant and maternal caregiver on the infant's structural brain development, and states that this "... indelibly set(s) the stage for every aspect of an organism's internal and external functioning throughout the lifespan"[14] (p. 3). This process takes place through the psychobiological regulation of neurohormones and catecholaminergic neurotransmitters in the infant's developing brain.[15] Predominance of a specific type of neurotransmitter may affect the specific structural development of areas of the developing brain.[16] The positive, symbiotic relationship experienced through closely attuned visual interaction between infant and mother regulates the neurochemistry of the infant's developing brain, and stimulates the development of pathways regulating positive affect states.[14] Schore also postulates that negative variations in this maternal-infant interaction during critical periods of growth and development of the infant's frontolimbic system can result in abnormal neuronal organization which in turn may contribute to the development of psychopathological behavioral patterns in adulthood.[17] In animal models, the continued survival of neuronal centers may be dependent on the repetition of appropriate facilitating experiences.[18] Studies of the structural development of the visual cortex in immature animals suggest that specific visual input and experience may be necessary for proper growth and function.[19,20] It is likely, therefore, that the developing brain is a fertile template for the laying-down of neuronal centers and synaptic connections formed on the basis of sensory input as part of complex early life experiences.

THE DEVELOPMENT OF CHARACTER

Grigsby and Hartlaub present another model of neural plasticity in the concept of formation of character as a function of procedural learning.[21] Procedural learning and memory, of course, refer to the processes of skill learning and conditioning, functions of nondeclarative, unconscious memory. "Character" may be defined as the exhibition of characteristic behavior in the face of specific internal and external stimuli, and probably is developed through repetitive experiential behavioral feedback sequences in infancy and childhood. Acquisition of information through this sequence is unconscious, and logically takes place through procedural memory mechanisms. Grigsby and Hartlaub maintain that, "This automatic, unconscious repeated performance of routine behaviors is the essence of character"[21] (p. 362). Since it is acquired through unconscious mechanisms, people are generally not aware of most of their individual character traits. In addition, procedural memories are by nature dissociable from declarative memories that are by definition largely conscious. As a result, determining the causes of character traits by logical analysis of historical events and their impact on the individual only provides an explanation, and does not change the unconscious, conditioned nature of the character trait.[22] Character, therefore, tends to remain very stable throughout life, changeable only through specific procedural learning that is directly related to procedurally acquired traits.

Many of the clinical characteristics of trauma also are associated with imprinting of events through procedural memory circuits.[23] Procedural learning associated with high emotional intensity—i.e., trauma—also has the capacity to produce significant character change, illustrating the plasticity of neuronal circuits that have been relatively "hard-wired" in childhood.[24] As a result, treatment approaches for both dysfunctional character traits and for PTSD logically will be extremely difficult if one uses techniques involving declarative memory and verbal interaction. Theoretically then, approaching procedural memory systems that determine the behavioral responses to specific events that determine character as well as traumatization might best be achieved through therapeutic techniques approaching unconscious memory through the autonomic or neuromuscular nervous systems. Such techniques are likely to involve the unconscious mechanisms of extinction, quenching, or desensitization, thereby bypassing the need for declarative memory or conscious and intentional imaging of the traumatic event.

BRAIN PLASTICITY IN TRAUMA

Numerous studies of autonomic and neuromuscular responses to trauma-related stimuli in PTSD patients suggest that relatively hard-wired changes in brain circuitry and response have occurred. Studies testing exposure of combat veterans to combat-related visual and auditory cues consistently show exaggerated heart rate, blood pressure, skin conductance, electromyography (EMG), and plasma epinephrine responses.[24] Based on these findings, Kolb has postulated that PTSD might be due to "conditioned emotional responses" similar to fear conditioning in animals.[26] The consistency of a conditioned response (autonomic reactivity) in combat veterans to a stereotyped conditioned stimulus (trauma-related memory cue) certainly supports this hypothesis.[24] This method of testing specific conditioned responses in trauma, however, is difficult to adapt to other types of trauma, such as child abuse, rape, accidents, or natural disasters. These sources of traumatic stress are often associated with more varied and complex conditioning stimuli, resulting in the procedural memory storage of diverse and often unpredictable traumatic cues.

Mental imagery should be quite adaptable as a conditioned stimulus to general populations of trauma victims. Studies of autonomic responsiveness to trauma-related mental imagery are reviewed again in Shalev and Rogel-Fuchs.[25] Predictably, combat veterans with PTSD show exaggerated autonomic response to combat-related imagery, whereas veterans without PTSD do not. Victims of sexual assault with PTSD show the same abnormal physiological traits, as do patients with MVA-related PTSD.[27] This response is dependent not just on exposure to the traumatic conditioning stimulus, but on whether clinical symptoms of PTSD resulted from that exposure. The consistency of an exaggerated autonomic response resulting from mental imagery also suggests a conditioned response to a conditioning stimulus, in this case a reminiscence. Pavlov, in fact, hypothesized the existence of a "secondary system of representation," involving memories, as well as verbal and visual images that were retained in memory. This "system" should be able to enhance learning and even conditioning without external sensory input.[28] This would fit with the concept of the kindled procedural memory/arousal/ neuromuscular feedback circuit discussed in Chapter 4.

In this model, declarative memory in the form of reminiscence serves as an additional trigger for the conditioned response. Diminishing traumatic arousal through extinction, therefore, might provide a means of reducing symptoms of PTSD if the input of reminiscence into the self-perpetuating neural circuit of PTSD could be reduced. Indeed, studies of repetitive imaginal exposure and even flooding have been found to reduce autonomic responsiveness to subsequent trauma-related imagery.[25,29] As one might expect, however, the contributions of declarative memory to the neural pathways serving traumatization appear easier to change through flooding than those served by procedural memory circuits that, in fact, may well be the major source of the contribution of memory to traumatic kindling. The measurable conditioned autonomic responses to an arousal stimulus noted in the previous studies tend to be the most permanently imprinted on procedural memory in trauma, and seem to be the most resistant to change with existing forms of therapy. Their persistence and constancy of expression suggest a neurophysiological and neurostructural change as permanent as that of character traits.

OBJECTIVE MEASURES OF BRAIN CHANGE IN TRAUMA

A permanent change in sympathetic physiological reactivity in patients suffering from chronic PTSD has been well documented in the literature. This also correlates with documented consistent cognitive changes in these patients, specifically in the area of verbal memory.[30] Further evidence for traumatic experience-based anatomic changes in brain structure have been documented with recent advances in brain imagery. Brain MRI studies suggest a significant reduction in hippocampal volume in Vietnam combat veterans suffering from PTSD.[31] Similar reduction in hippocampal volume has been documented in female victims of childhood sexual abuse.[32]

High serum levels of serum cortisol have been implicated in this effect on the hippocampus in both human and animal studies, both in vivo and in vitro. Activation of the hypothalamic/pituitary/adrenal axis (HPA) as part of the initial adaptive hormonal response to stress results in prolonged elevation of levels of glucocorticoids in the body. Although glucocorticoids are crucial in modulating the acute response to stress initiated by norepinephrine, prolonged exposure to elevated levels of these hormones results in damage to hippocampal neurons, both in the in vitro rat brain,[33] and in vivo studies in primates.[34] Prolonged exposure to stress in primates also has been shown to cause selective hippocampal damage.[35] These findings of experience-based anatomical changes in brain structure are quite consistent with theories previously cited by Schore.[14]

Another example of dynamic changes in regional brain structure and function has been noted using positron emission tomography (PET) associated with exposure of traumatized individuals to detailed narratives related to their trauma.[36] While patients read arousing personal narratives, PET scans were taken of their brains. Localized increased metabolic activity was uniformly documented in the right hemisphere in the specific region in the limbic system associated with the amygdala—the region of the brain serving memory associated with arousal and anxiety. Increased activity in the right visual cortex was consistent with the presence of flashbacks experienced during the study. Interestingly, Broca's area for speech showed reduced activity, consistent with the symptom of *alexithymia,* the inability of PTSD patients to express emotions in words.[36] Similar scans of individuals without PTSD did not show this pattern, indicating the existence of a persistent change in regional brain function in PTSD.

The cingulate gyrus plays an important role in the brain's physiological response to threat as part of the limbic system, and demonstrates predictable changes in blood flow during fear activation in PTSD. The anterior cingulate serves an inhibitory gating function on fear conditioning by the amygdala, and also plays a role in generation of maternal behavior and social bonding. The posterior cingulate helps regulate processing of visual images, a function important in processing of information regarding threatening events, as evidenced by right visual cortical enhancement during traumatic imagery in PTSD.[36] PET studies during exposure to traumatic stimuli in PTSD show a failure of activation of the anterior cingulate,[37,38] consistent with sustained inhibition of the gating control of the amygdala in PTSD, a persistent change in brain physiology that might contribute to perpetuation of arousal-based kindling. The role of the anterior cingulate in the development of PTSD and dissociation will be discussed further in Chapter 8.

THE PERMANENCE
OF POST-TRAUMATIC STRESS DISORDER

Longitudinal studies of patients with PTSD show evidence not only for chronicity, but for actual decline in standard measures of personal and social functioning.[39] This deterioration would be in keeping with the model of PTSD as self-perpetuated kindling involving brain centers associated with memory and arousal, and closely linked to avoidance and the dysfunctional phenomenon of dissociation. It would also be in keeping with permanent changes in neuronal interaction that would restrict the behavioral options of the traumatized individual. Based on the verified relationship of prolonged glucocorticoid exposure to permanent changes in hippocampal structure and function, one would expect this effect to contribute to a sequential decline in functional coping skills in the victim of PTSD. Surprisingly, studies of urinary free-cortisol levels in those patients with late or chronic PTSD show low, stable levels when compared to patients with other types of psychopathology.[40]

In addition, these chronic PTSD patients demonstrate relative elevation of urinary norepinephrine levels, resulting in an unusual elevation of the norepinephrine/cortisol ratio.[41] This is in contrast to the well-established elevation of both norepinephrine and cortisol in acute stress. One explanation for this unusual late suppression of serum cortisol in late PTSD might be that adaptive mechanisms to the continuously kindled arousal of PTSD might suppress rather than stimulate the HPA axis without suppressing adrenergic arousal. Several studies have shown that certain psychological defense mechanisms, especially denial, can powerfully suppress urinary cortisol levels, both chronically,[42] and even lower in acute stress.[43] The possibility that adrenal cortical exhaustion explained the suppression of low chronic cortisol levels in PTSD was ruled out in one of these studies by the administration of adrenocorticosteroid hormone, and the production of a normal cortisol response.[44] Cortisol, therefore, seems to exhibit a paradoxical role in acute traumatic stress versus late PTSD, suggesting that the evolution of the posttraumatic syndrome is associated with basic changes in the core physiology of the brain and the body.

On a psychodynamic basis, denial and dissociation share many similarities. Dissociation is one of the cardinal features of the late adaptive mechanisms of PTSD. Dissociation at the time of traumatization correlates with later development of PTSD more than any other measured variable.[45] Those individuals who dissociate at the time of the trauma will tend to dissociate under later conditions of stress, especially if the initial trauma was in childhood (see Chapter 8). The neurochemical substrate of dissociation has not been well established, although the numbing and constriction associated with many of its features suggest endorphinergic and perhaps serotinergic mechanisms. The persistence of dissociation in chronic PTSD may play a role in suppression of the HPA axis, and contribute to the loss of adaptation to the continued cyclical arousal in chronic PTSD. Suppression of serum cortisol in these patients in that model would prevent the modulating effect of glucocorticoids on the acute effects of epinephrine, serving to perpetuate the seemingly permanent neurophysiological changes of this condition. These theoretical considerations, and the role of the parasympathetic nervous system in PTSD will be explored in more detail in Chapter 8.

CONCLUSION

Exposure to stress, trauma, and the process of traumatization has profound effects on the brain and the endocrine system, especially the HPA axis. This effect is crucial for the initial neuroendocrine response to a threatening event, but soon begins to have deleterious and ultimately long-standing effects on neuronal structure and function. Imaging studies of the brain, both anatomical and functional, suggest that this effect is long-lasting and in some instances probably permanent. The implications of this data with regards to the effectiveness of therapy for PTSD, and the likelihood of achieving a cure for its disabling symptoms are grave.

The concept of kindling as a source of development and perpetuation of the neurophysiological basis for PTSD is quite consistent with the permanence of PTSD. Kindling also provides a theoretical basis for the possibility of associated permanent anatomical and physiological neuronal change in traumatic stress. These concepts are also in keeping with emerging theories addressing the hardwired experiential basis for brain development, the development of character, and the vulnerability to psychopathology. Thus far, the elusive changes in brain function seen in imaging studies, as well as the contradictory findings in HPA axis function in victims of trauma, appear to be the

Chapter 6

Diseases of Traumatic Stress

Pat had been involved in a relatively minor but particularly terrifying auto accident. While stopped at a light behind a large dump truck, the truck inexplicably began to back up. Unable to retreat due to the car behind her, and apparently unseen by the truck driver, she watched in horror as the truck slowly bore down on her, and slowly crushed the hood and engine compartment of her car. Her car was shaken, but not moved, and the noise of the crushing of metal finally prompted the truck driver to stop. Pat was predictably shocked, stunned, and numb, and took hours to recover her senses and awareness of what had happened to her.

Thereafter, she developed headaches, neck pain, panic attacks, and full-blown post-traumatic stress disorder, along with significant cognitive problems. Within a week of the accident, she developed influenza, with a severe eruption of herpes labialis. She missed her next menstrual period, and within six weeks, gained twelve pounds, with most of the weight embarrassingly concentrated about her waist. Several bladder infections followed in the ensuing months, and heartburn and symptoms of gastroesophageal reflux prompted a diagnostic workup by a gastroenterologist, with negative results. As her neck pain worsened and spread to her low back, shoulders, and arms, she noted increasing morning stiffness, and generalized pain and sensitivity to touch. Combined with interrupted, nonrestorative sleep and chronic fatigue, she was ultimately diagnosed by a rheumatologist as suffering from fibromyalgia, chronic fatigue syndrome, and irritable bowel syndrome. A physician who performed an independent medical examination for her automobile insurance company, however, concluded that she was probably suffering from conversion and somatization, and that secondary gain issues must be considered,

since the accident itself was certainly negligible with regard to the
possibility of significant physical injury.

* * *

THE PATHOPHYSIOLOGY OF STRESS

The concept that prolonged or excessive exposure to stress could
contribute to the development of specific diseases was formulated by
Selye in 1936.[1] His original studies are mentioned in Chapter 2, and
have led to the conclusion that exposure of the organism to a variety
of stressors would result in a complex neuroendocrine response primarily involving the hormones of the pituitary and adrenal cortex.
These responses were critical to the survival of the organism when
subjected to an acute stress, but exposure to prolonged or cumulative
stress could result in damage to the organism, much of which correlated with prolonged exposure to adrenal cortical hormones. Thus
rats subjected to prolonged, inescapable stress were found to develop
erosion of the gastric mucosa, atherosclerosis, and adrenal cortical atrophy. More than a half century of research stimulated by his findings
has served to validate them, and to support the role of pituitary/adre-
nal cortical activity in stress modulation.

The role of cortisol and other glucocorticoids in modulating the
acute role of norepinephrine in stress has been discussed (Chapter 4).
Cortisol modulates the acute effects of norepinephrine-induced arousal on limbic structures in response to acute stress. Cortisol also acts to
regulate the hypothalamic/pituitary/adrenal axis in the ongoing response to stress via a negative feedback loop to the hypothalamus and
pituitary gland. The complex, multisystemic effects of gluco- and
mineralocorticoids also serve to manage the body's secondary line of
defense to stress. These effects include sodium retention with increased intravascular volume, mobilization of hepatic glycogen and
increased insulin secretion, mobilization of calcium from bone stores,
increase in lipogenesis, increase in peptic acid secretion, suppression
of lymphocyte formation, and cerebral cortical stimulation. The resulting immune, metabolic, and neuronal responses are important in the
organism's early defenses to abnormal stressors, but if prolonged,
may lead to specific organ damage.

The resulting "diseases of stress" reflect the well-known systemic side effects of prolonged therapeutic glucocorticoid administration. These diseases include diabetes, atherosclerosis, hypertension, peptic ulcer disease, obesity, osteoporosis, and cognitive/emotional impairment. In addition, selective regional patterns of neuronal death primarily involving the hippocampus have been documented in many studies of animals subjected to prolonged exposure to cortisol (see Chapter 5). These diseases appear to accurately reflect the findings in Selye's chronically stressed rats. Clearly, chronic and prolonged exposure to unremitting life stress is associated with a cluster of vascular, hormonal, immunological, neuronal, and degenerative diseases that are largely attributable to exposure to abnormal amounts of glucocorticoids.

STRESS VERSUS TRAUMA

Prolonged stress and trauma, although basically part of the same continuum, differ in a number of ways. Stress may be defined in one sense as any negative stimulus that produces activation of the sympathetic nervous system and related HPA pathways. Trauma may be viewed in this light as an extreme form of stress, one that has assumed life-threatening proportions. Trauma also is usually a sentinel event or events of great threat and magnitude, eliciting a maximal catecholamine-based arousal. On the other hand, trauma need not be *traumatizing* unless, as defined in the DSM-IV, it elicits a behavioral response of fear, horror, or a sense of helplessness, a state very suggestive of elements of the freeze/immobility response.

In our previous discussion of the meaning of the freeze response, and the role of the lack of completion of the freeze discharge in the development of PTSD, we noted that the physiology of freezing involves intense parasympathetic tone. This physiological state represents a temporary adaptation to acute stress that is not physiologically sustainable, and one that is certainly not associated with continued adrenergic arousal and elevation of serum cortisol. As we have noted, the freeze response very likely is associated with the phenomenon of dissociation, an event that is a powerful predictor of the subsequent development of PTSD in individuals subjected to a traumatic experience. Traumatic stress and the development of PTSD are not inevitable with exposure to stress or trauma, however life-threatening. These events very likely depend on the event of the freeze/immobility response occurring in a state of helplessness associated with that threat, and perhaps on the perpetuation of dissociation as a secondary event. One might therefore expect to see a substantial difference in the biological changes that occur in chronic stress, trauma, and traumatic stress.

THE HYPOTHALAMIC/ PITUITARY/ADRENAL AXIS

Unlike Selye's model of diseases of stress associated with prolonged exposure to abnormal levels of glucocorticoids, patients with PTSD exhibit hormonal changes suggestive of abnormal function of the hypothalamic/pituitary/adrenal (HPA) axis. If you will recall, input to the hypothalamus from the locus ceruleus as a result of an arousal stimulus triggers release of corticotropin-releasing hormone (CRH), which in turn stimulates release of adrenocorticotropic hormone (ACTH) by the pituitary. ACTH stimulates the release of cortisol by the adrenal cortex, which in turn modulates the effect of norepinephrine-mediated messages within the brain, thereby controlling the arousal reflex. One would expect levels of serum cortisol to be elevated therefore in acute stress, as in Selye's model of stress-related disease. Studies of serum cortisol in late stage or chronic PTSD, however, show abnormally low levels of serum cortisol and twenty-four-hour urinary cortisol excretion.[2,3,4] In addition, binding sites for cortisol in the brain and on lymphocytes normally tend to increase with low serum levels of glucocorticoids. Therefore, it is not surprising in late PTSD, where serum cortisol is low, that increased numbers of lymphocyte glucocorticoid receptors were also found.[3] This apparent paradox is contradictory to previously noted concepts of the role of cortisol as a modulator of trauma-induced epinephrine release, and of the response of the HPA axis to traumatic stress. It does suggest, however, that the HPA axis is somehow sensitized in PTSD.

Further evidence for a sensitized HPA axis in chronic PTSD is found in the Dexamethasone Suppression Test (DST). Administration of dexamethasone in the normal individual suppresses release of CRH by the hypothalamus as well as adrenocorticotropic hormone (ACTH) by the pituitary, since dexamethasone mimics the inhibitory effect of cortisol on the HPA axis. As a result, by inhibiting the HPA axis, dexamethasone secondarily inhibits cortisol release by the adrenal cortex by substituting for the patient's own cortisol, thereby "fooling" the HPA axis into shutting down. Chronic PTSD patients actually show an exaggerated suppression of cortisol release with the DST, again suggesting a highly sensitized HPA axis in these patients.[5] In addition, impairment of the release of ACTH by the pituitary is noted in PTSD patients in response to an overstimulating exposure to hypothalamic CRH.[6] This is further evidence for HPA dysfunction in this group of patients.

Admittedly these findings are far from conclusive in defining the abnormal stress response in PTSD. They do, however, tend to separate PTSD from other psychiatric conditions with regard to their relationship to the sympathetic nervous system, the HPA axis, and the more traditional model of the stress response developed by Selye.[7] They also may have implications regarding the unique spectrum of diseases that may accompany chronic symptoms of PTSD.

STRESS, POST-TRAUMATIC STRESS DISORDER, AND IMMUNE FUNCTION

Alteration of the immune system has been one of the more thoroughly studied examples of the health effects of inordinate stress. Studies of the effects of stress on viral immunity have generally shown consistently increased vulnerability to infection. Cold virus inoculations in unstressed subjects and in those exposed to stress have shown increased vulnerability to respiratory infection in the stressed subjects.[8] Antibody levels to Epstein-Barr virus (EBV), hepatitis B virus, herpes simplex virus, and cytomegalovirus have been noted to consistently rise with stress.[9,10,11] Increased viral antibody titers in these cases represent reduced cellular immunity, indicating immune suppression. Immune responses to stress in human immunodeficiency virus (HIV) in limited studies show that stress may induce reduction of total lymphocytes and natural killer cells.[12,13] Clearly, exposure to high levels of chronic stress may increase susceptibility to infectious diseases due to immune suppression.

Natural killer (NK) cells constitute a main line of defense by the immune system against not only infectious agents, but also mutated cancer cells. In acute stress, elevation of epinephrine (E) and norepinephrine (NE) as part of the fight/flight response is associated with increased NK cell activity. The fact that this increase in immune function is directly due to effects of E and NE on an acute basis is supported by the fact that the increase of NK activity in these cases is blocked by propranolol. Propranalol is a peripheral beta-adrenergic blocker, and therefore an inhibitor of peripheral effects of epinephrine.[14] It has also long been known that high levels of cortisol associated with early responses to trauma and stress impair immune function, hence the long-standing use of synthetic forms of cortisol in organ transplants in order to inhibit immune rejection of the organ.

By contrast, *chronic* exposure to stress results in reduction in NK cell activity despite continued increase in E and NE levels.[15] In addition, exposure to chronic stress actually inhibits the increased NK activity response to acute stress.[16] Exposure to chronic stress therefore appears to inhibit one of the body's frontline immune defenses, and to inhibit the natural increase in immune defenses in the face of new and acute stress. The clinical effects of chronic stress on viral infections would certainly suggest that stress-induced immune suppression is clinically significant with regard to general health. Therefore, one would expect relative immune suppression and vulnerability to infectious disease in acute PTSD, where serum cortisol is also elevated. In *chronic* PTSD victims, however, serum cortisol levels tend to be low, a state where the modulating effect of cortisol on the immune system is decreased. Under these circumstances, the biological effects of late PTSD might facilitate immune activity, and contribute to vulnerability to autoimmune diseases. Meaningful data with regard to the theoretical increased risk of cancer or other immune deficiency diseases related to stress-induced impairment of the immune response, and increased risk of autoimmune disease to lower serum cortisol levels in chronic PTSD, is unfortunately not available at this time. A clue to this possible relationship, however, may be found in epidemiological studies of the incidence of chronic disease in populations of patients who have been exposed to prolonged and severe traumatic stress.

THE DISEASES OF TRAUMA

Chronic Pain

One of the most studied symptoms associated with prior histories of severe trauma is chronic pain. Many of these studies address the effects of childhood abuse on chronic pain complaints, especially in women sexually abused in childhood. The baseline incidence of childhood sexual abuse in women has been estimated at anywhere from 12 to 64 percent of the general female population in various studies.[17-22] The average probably falls somewhere around 30 percent. In males, the incidence is predictably less that half of that figure. Many studies document the association between childhood physical and sexual abuse and chronic pain. Perhaps the most well-studied association is that between female childhood sexual abuse and chronic pelvic pain.[23-29] In general, these studies show a significantly higher incidence of childhood sexual abuse in women with medically unexplained pelvic pain than controls or comparison groups, such as women seeking tubal ligation. Other studies, however, show that childhood physical abuse predicted all adult pain syndromes as well or better than sexual abuse.[30] Taken together, childhood sexual, physical, and psychological abuse are powerful predictors of chronic pelvic, abdominal, low back, orofacial, and myofascial pain.[31-35]

Comorbidity of epidemiological events, of course, does not prove a cause-and-effect association. One must find a common rationale for this relationship on a solid theoretical basis, combined with the weight of controlled scientific studies to arrive at a justified etiological conclusion. Obviously, this goal is not within the scope of this book. I believe, however, that the core concept of the neurophysiology of PTSD and its relationship to the basic features of the whiplash syndrome allow us to expand concepts of perpetuation of symptoms of many chronic diseases, especially chronic pain.

Classical operant conditioning as a basic feature of implicit memory is a key to the understanding of this concept. Conditioning is not a laboratory phenomenon, but is the key system of information access responsible for individual and species survival. Conditioned responses to an identifiable life threat must take place in one or two trials, or else the specific gene matrix of the unfortunate prey animal is discarded, probably for the betterment of the species. Sensory information for all of the experiences associated with that life threat is incorporated immediately, and hopefully forever, into the implicit memory of the surviving animal for future reference and application in a similar threatening situation. In the example of myofascial pain after an MVA, I believe that the proprioceptive memory of the protective movements of the body in the accident generated by stretch receptors are immediately and indelibly stored in brainstem motor centers. Thereafter, they will be resurrected time and again in situations of perceived life threat, leading to recurrent regional patterns of myo-fascial pain. This event by definition assumes that a truncated freeze response has contributed to the late phenomenon of kindled arousal/ memory circuitry, with the patterns of motor memory stored in the kindled loop of PTSD. In other words, the reflex-bracing pattern of those specific muscle groups has a *meaning* in terms of survival to those centers of the brain responsible for this function. Nociceptive pain associated with structural somatic injury, occurring in the same context of a life threat without freeze resolution, will continue to be incorporated within implicit memory in situations of threat in order to facilitate the "survival brain" in its instinctual goals. Until that pain no longer represents a message about the unresolved threat, it will continue to be recycled into conscious awareness to protect the trau-matized creature/individual in situations of cue-related, or eventually nonspecific arousal. The dramatic incidence of prior life trauma, and the traumatic origins of pain in those patients treated in chronic pain programs is well known. This fact is also in keeping with the previous concept: the incorporation of meaningful pain messages into proce-dural and implicit sensorimotor memory in the process of traumatic kindling is a contributing cause of persisting pain in the apparent ab-sence of tissue pathology. This concept is in keeping with well-known but poorly understood phenomena of chronic pain such as phantom limb pain.

Reflex Sympathetic Dystrophy

Concepts of chronic regional myofascial and somatic pain may well apply to the development of many chronic regional pain syndromes through similar mechanisms. Obviously, sympathetically maintained pain presents an intriguing possibility as an example of traumatically facilitated chronic regional pain. Reflex sympathetic dystrophy (RSD) was first described in the context of wounds suffered on the battle-field.[36] Although RSD has been associated with a bewildering va-riety of conditions, the majority of precipitating events are associated with a traumatic event (fractures, dislocations, wounds, traumatic neuropathies, soft tissue injuries, strokes, acute radiculopathies).[37,38]

The syndrome is associated with a variety of classic symptoms and findings, a majority of which consist of vasomotor symptoms suggestive of autonomic dysregulation of the involved region of the body. Burning, hyperpathic pain, and allodynia are the hallmark symptoms, and early vasomotor signs may present as warm, red, and dry skin, or conversely as cool and pale skin, with diaphoresis. Trophic changes with increased hair and nail growth may be seen in the early stages. Later, dystrophic or atrophic changes may occur, involving hypothermia, regional osteoporosis, hair and nail loss, skin and muscle atrophy, edema, dystonia, and joint contractures. Personality characteristics have been studied in victims of RSD, and early reports have described RSD patients as "hypersympathetic reactors," with behavioral traits of insecurity, lability, and anxiety. Specific studies, however, have failed to document premorbid psychological disturbances in RSD patients, but also have failed to investigate childhood abuse or prior trauma history in these patients.[39,40]

The syndrome varies widely in severity and the number of clinical signs that accompany it, leading to attempts to break down the classification into subsets such as sympathetically maintained pain and complex regional pain syndrome. The typical vasomotor signs primarily suggest a role for increased peripheral sympathetic activity in the pathology of this condition. In addition, the variable positive therapeutic response to sympathetic ganglia blockade through infusion of the alpha-adrenergic blocker, phentolamine, or through sympathetic ganglia blockade by direct injection, have implicated excessive activity of the sympathetic nervous system in the etiology. Specific oculocephalic sympathetic dysfunction in the form of bilateral postganglionic Horner's syndrome and supraorbital anhydrosis has been documented in cases of posttraumatic headache.[41] As an aside, altered autonomic vasomotor functions that might produce these types of clinical signs suggest that posttraumatic headache in general may have its roots in autonomic dysfunction related to RSD.

On the other hand, the variability of response to therapy and the inconsistency of clinical presentation have cast some doubt on the specificity of the role of sympathetic dysfunction in RSD as a primary cause. Sensory findings in the neurological examination, although occasionally representative of a peripheral nerve or nerve root distribution, usually assume a stocking/glove, or other nonanatomical distribution after the syndrome has been present for some time.

Both peripheral and central neuropathological mechanisms have been proposed, with a central nervous system cause being perhaps more appealing due to the well-documented though rare cases of spread of the syndrome to other regions of the body, and occasionally to bilateral involvement. Fortunately, remission and disappearance of symptoms and signs in mild cases is common. Linking RSD to trauma is tempting for several reasons. In many cases, RSD is a direct progression of a specific traumatic injury, as in a war or accident-related wound. Both sympathetic and parasympathetic physiological and pathological manifestations accompany the syndrome. Behavioral and personality variations are commonly associated with RSD. Many features, including sensory symptoms atypical for a peripheral etiology and spread of the condition in a physiologically atypical pattern, suggest a central etiology. Kindled implicit memory for pain in the face of unresolved trauma, autonomic dysregulation in PTSD, and the traumatic origin of RSD in many cases make a strong circumstantial case for this bizarre syndrome to be linked to the existing neurophysiological models of PTSD. As we shall see in Chapter 8, I believe that RSD is in fact much more than that, and may present a prototype for many of the unresolved challenges of the somatic manifestations and disorders associated with PTSD.

Fibromyalgia/Chronic Fatigue Syndrome

Another common chronic pain syndrome that may have its roots in traumatization is fibromyalgia. First described by Gowers in 1904,[42] it has been exhaustively investigated in numerous, generally flawed studies, and has remained as controversial as one might expect of a syndrome with remarkably uniform and reproducible symptoms, but with few if any objective signs. Clinical criteria for the diagnosis are generally based on consistency of symptoms and the presence of at least seven "tender points" in specific areas over the surface of the body. Typical symptoms include multiple regional or diffuse sites of soft tissue pain, poor and nonrestorative sleep, chronic fatigue, stiffness, headaches, irritable bowel syndrome, anxiety, cognitive dysfunction, and variable neurological symptoms, especially numbness and paresthesia. These symptoms typically are aggravated by stress, weather changes, and physical activity.

Another syndrome closely linked to fibromyalgia, with similar symptoms except for the absence of soft tissue pain, is chronic fatigue syndrome (CFS). In addition to many other similar symptoms, fibromyalgia and CFS share similar sleep disturbances. The EEG pattern during sleep in fibromyalgia and CFS is characterized by abnormal presence of alpha (7.5 to 11 Hz) wave activity seen during deeper non-REM cycles of sleep. This EEG pattern is consistent with a recurrent nonphysiological arousal disturbance, and coincides with the repeated nocturnal awakening characteristic of fibromyalgia and CFS. Interestingly, this unusual EEG pattern is also typical of the arousal disturbance seen in myofascial pain, PTSD, ambient nocturnal noise, and painful joint disease in rheumatoid arthritis.[43]

The clinical syndromes of fibromyalgia and CFS have remarkable similarities to those symptoms affecting whiplash victims with delayed recovery, and the later symptom complex of chronic PTSD (see Chapter 3). I have followed several whiplash patients who over several years have eventually progressed from regional myofascial pain to clinically consistent criteria-specific generalized fibromyalgia. All members of this group of patients had experienced childhood trauma except for one rape victim. Posttraumatic fibromyalgia has been reported in numerous studies, and generally follows soft tissue injuries. One study of 176 cases of posttraumatic fibromyalgia documented that 60.7 percent occurred after MVAs, 12.5 percent after work-related injuries, 7.1 percent after surgery, 5.4 percent after sports-related injury, and 14.3 percent after miscellaneous traumatic events.[44] The majority of these events represent substantial trauma in the face of helplessness.

Neuroendocrine changes in fibromyalgia also suggest a traumatic link. Studies of the HPA axis in fibromyalgia and CFS show remarkably similar aberrations to those seen in PTSD. These changes include low basal twenty-four-hour urine cortisol excretion, blunted cortisol circadian rhythms, exaggerated ACTH response to CRH, and a blunted cortisol response to increased ACTH.[45] The HPA axis in CFS also reveals lowered basal cortisol levels, and an attenuated ACTH response to CRH, as seen in PTSD.[46] Depressed pituitary insulin-like growth factor (IGF-I) has been documented in those patients with fibromyalgia, and gives further evidence for HPA dysfunction.[47] Finally, hypervigilance to a variety of external and internal noxious sensations, including pain, has been documented in fibromyalgia.[48,49] Hypervigilence and nonspecific stimulus sensitivity, of course, are intrinsic to the diagnosis of PTSD. This association, not surprisingly, has attracted a great deal of scientific attention, leading to scores of articles studying the related incidence of childhood physical and sexual abuse in cases of fibromyalgia. Typical reports of the incidence of incest in fibromyalgia patients reveal figures varying from 37 to 65 percent, compared to control group incidence varying from 42 to 52 percent.[50,51] (Perhaps the most shocking figure in these studies is the incidence of childhood sexual abuse in the control groups!) Retrospective studies such as these, of course, are vulnerable to bias on the part of the respondents, as well as to the problems associated with attributing a causative relationship to consistently coexistent life events.

Nevertheless, many clinical and physiological clues appear to link fibromyalgia/CFS to a traumatic etiology. The predominance of fibromyalgia and CFS in women (>75 percent), the gender prevalence of sexual and physical abuse in women, and the tendency for women to dissociate with trauma and to develop typical PTSD (see Chapter 8) place them at greater risk for both conditions. Similar hormonal markers, arousal sensitivity, and symptom complexes of fibromyalgia/CFS and PTSD demand consideration for an etiological relationship between trauma and the fibromyalgia/CFS syndrome.

Somatization Disorders

Symptoms defined as somatization disorders are not surprisingly extremely common in child abuse survivors. Adults who have suffered physical and sexual abuse as children have a substantially higher incidence than control groups of functional gastrointestinal disorders, genitourinary symptoms and lifetime surgical procedures, most of which did not cure the symptom, or in which no pathology was found.[32,52,53] Somatization in psychiatric terms actually refers to a tendency to express painful emotions as physical symptoms in traumatized patients, possibly related to the inability of such patients to remember traumatic memory in a verbal context. Abuse histories for patients in these studies also correlated with greater symptom complaints in general, and greater utilization of health care services. This fact would certainly be consistent with the tendency for somatization to occur in traumatized individuals. A predominance of visceral complaints in these victims would certainly be consistent with their vulnerability to recurrent arousal, autonomic dysregulation, and dissociation. I believe that somatization and conversion represent more than an aberration of pain memory based on trauma. Regional and systemic somatization symptoms and signs of conversion may well represent measurable pathophysiological changes that are associated with objective disease processes in the symptomatic end organs (see Chapter 8).

At the same time, abuse victims frequently do not report their abuse history to their treating physician. Probably 20 to 50 percent of episodes of abuse are unreported, both at the time and later in life,[54] suggesting that the incidence of child abuse in somatization syndromes may be much higher than current estimates. In addition, I believe that the definition of what specifically constitutes a "traumatic life event" is based to a significant event on cultural bias, gender-specific definitions, and a general lack of understanding of the physiological tolerance to stress of the developing infant. Added to this dilemma is the well-documented tendency for a society to deny its social ills, as exemplified by Freud's recanting of his theories of incest and conversion hysteria under pressure from his peers, as addressed in Chapter 5.

The incidence and cost of diagnostic and therapeutic surgical procedures, including laparoscopies, cystoscopies, colonoscopies, and hysterectomies related to these traumatically based functional complaints has not been accurately documented. Walker and colleagues, however, have estimated that the *annual* medical cost per childhood abuse survivor for symptoms related to somatization averages $4,700.[28] Upon completion of the expensive, essentially normal diagnostic evaluation for a somatization-based complaint, the physician will be reassuring, but will often justifiably address the possible "psychological" basis for the complaint. The somatization patients, unable to express emotion other than by physical symptoms, will be further devalued and traumatized by the denial of the physical validity of their very real pain, and not surprisingly, will continue to pursue the elusive symptom to the frustration of their medical providers.

MORBIDITY AND MORTALITY

In addition to increased reporting of symptoms and increased use of medical services, victims of trauma also experience increased morbidity and mortality rates.[55] Studies have tended to focus on war-related trauma, with many of them addressing health status of former prisoners of war (POWs).[56,57] Many of these former POWs experienced increased gastrointestinal and cardiovascular complaints and illnesses, especially peptic ulcer disease, hypertension, and myocardial infarction. In addition, increased mortality was noted in these POWs, especially in the areas of accidents, suicide, and cirrhosis of the liver.[58] These mortality statistics, of course, could be related to the emotional sequelae of war trauma, and the associated increased incidence of alcohol abuse. Cardiovascular morbidity and mortality, however, appear to be more specific complications of wartime stress as documented in the above studies, and in studies of residents of Lebanon and Croatia during civil wars in those countries.[59,60] In cases of childhood abuse, however, the literature is less clear regarding increased incidence of disease processes in adulthood. Most of the problems experienced in adult survivors of child abuse seem to fall into the classification of functional diseases rather than objective organic disease.[53] Felitti and colleagues, however, have recently documented a strong graded relationship between the degree and severity of exposure to abuse or dysfunctional family behavior patterns during childhood and a number of the leading causes of death during adulthood.[61] This study provides convincing evidence for the dangers of unresolved traumatic stress to one's health and life, especially trauma experienced during childhood.

When the clinical diagnosis of PTSD is added to the equation, however, the incidence and significance of adverse health effects of trauma increases significantly.[55,62] The greatest area of vulnerability probably involves the cardiovascular system,[63,64] a predictable association considering the cardiovascular effects of the stress and fight/flight responses. Specific studies of the cardiovascular effects of sympathetic autonomic dysregulation in primates certainly support the concept of a role of stress in the development of atherosclerotic cardiovascular disease.[65]

In their review of the relationship between stress, PTSD, and health, Friedman and Schnurr hypothesize that the widespread changes induced by the neurochemical substrate of PTSD have significant adverse health effects.[55] Hypertension and atherosclerotic cardiovascular disease are likely among the most common and obvious effects of autonomic dysregulation. Endocrinological abnormalities, especially HPA dysregulation and altered thyroid function, not only may lead to specific endocrine disturbances, but also to immune disorders. Suppression of the immune system by initial HPA activation and hypercortisolemia might increase susceptibility to infection, as noted earlier in this chapter. Conversely, lowered serum cortisol levels documented in chronic, late stage PTSD might be expected to produce increased immune activation. Alteration in the genetic phenotypes of blood lymphocytes in PTSD indeed suggests the potentiation of increased immune activation.[66] Other authors have also postulated that immune dysregulation might also predispose PTSD victims to autoimmune disorders.[55]

CONCLUSION

Although much of the scientific data associating traumatic stress with adverse health effects is circumstantial and subject to debate and interpretation, many studies show physiological alterations in PTSD that correlate with predictable diseases seen in its victims. There also appears to be a small cluster of poorly understood syndromes that have a compelling link to the physiology and incidence of trauma, including irritable bowel syndrome, interstitial cystitis, chronic pain syndromes, fibromyalgia/CFS, and RSD. Other so-called diseases of stress, including hypertension, peptic ulcer disease, ulcerative colitis, and atherosclerotic coronary artery disease probably also can be added to the list of diseases of trauma. Idiopathic autoimmune syndromes need to be considered as well. Because the physiological events associated with stress and trauma are by nature fluctuating and dynamic, consistent measurement of these events in relationship to clinical symptoms or signs remains a challenge. Proof of a direct relationship between trauma and these syndromes therefore is likely to be extremely difficult. The evidence at hand also suggests that stress and trauma alone are often not sufficient to cause these diseases. The physiological event of traumatic stress or freeze/dissociation appears to be an important element in triggering the required pathological events. Since the autonomic nervous system in PTSD may well be associated with the self-perpetuating central nervous system phenomenon of kindling, it is likely that the resulting continuous perturbation of vascular, endocrinological, and immune systems is required to contribute to the development of these diseases of trauma. As diseases of kindling, one might expect them to progress in severity in the apparent absence of an ongoing identifiable pathogenic event. The remarkable prevalence of trauma in modern society is amply demonstrated in the PTSD literature. In this model, therefore, the pathophysiological effects of trauma might well provide the major impetus to development and perpetuation of many chronic diseases of unknown cause. A more specific rationale for this relationship will be developed in Chapter 8, linking the process of dissociation to pathological autonomic dysregulation, leading to regional vasomotor disease in the dissociated end organ.

Finally, the distinction between the "psychological" and physical pathological manifestations of traumatic stress, as suggested in the term "psychosomatic," needs to be discarded. The pathophysiological, neurobiological, endocrinological, and immunological changes induced by trauma form a continuum with the subsequent pathological somatic manifestations of disease. Based on Weiner's[67,68] and Grotstein's[69] observations, Schore[70] states: "Weiner's fundamental understanding that all physical disease represents a disturbance of regulation and Grotstein's penetrating insight that all psychopathology represents disordered self-regulation clearly indicate that a differentiation between physical and psychosomatic disease is meaningless and misleading." The trauma therefore changes the brain, which therefore changes the body.

Chapter 7

Trauma Reenactment

Tracey was injured when she was knocked off of her bike in a cross-walk by a car that was making a right turn. When I evaluated her two weeks later, she appeared to have suffered only soft tissue injuries, but also was experiencing a great deal of hyperarousal, irritability, stimulus sensitivity, and sleep disturbance. I prescribed some physical therapy as well as a course of Eye Movement Desensitization and Reprocessing (EMDR) to deal with her residual subsyndromal PTSD.

The accident occurred on January 26. On March 26, she lost control of her car on a mountain road and narrowly escaped going over the edge. On May 26, while bending over to pick something up, her room-mate's dog leaped up, hit her in her left eye, and blackened the eye. On June 26, she severely sprained her right ankle. At that point, she realized that something strange was happening, and came back to see me. She told me that toward the end of each month, she had developed a sense of depression and foreboding without her actually recalling the accident. Upon looking at her calendar, she was astonished to note that each subsequent accident had occurred on the same day of the month as her original bicycle mishap.

* * *

INTRODUCTION

Victims of traumatization live in a perpetually altered state of response to stress and arousal. Vietnam veterans suffering from PTSD continue to produce dramatically elevated levels of adrenaline when exposed to a stimulus related to their past traumatic memories, such as the noise of a helicopter flying overhead or the smell of oriental food.[1] When exposed to scenes of warfare in a video, their brains not only produce more adrenaline, but also release increased amounts of endorphins, the pain-modulating neurotransmitters, or messengers. Testing their pain thresholds at that time showed reduced pain perception even as they were experiencing significant arousal. As far back as World War II, researchers documented that acutely wounded soldiers seemed to require less morphine for pain relief than one would expect from the severity of their injuries.[2] There are many anecdotes of soldiers with painful injuries continuing to fight in the heat of battle, seemingly ignoring their pain. We suspect that endorphins released at times of great stress and threat to life, as well as in situations of great physical exertion, serve to dampen pain perception in order to allow maximal survival effort.[3] Attention to ones' wounds in an acute survival emergency could well impede survival behavior. Not surprisingly, therefore, endorphins appear to play a pivotal role in not only the early, but also the late behavioral characteristics of traumatized individuals. This phenomenon of pain modulation in stress by endorphins may contribute to one of the more bizarre and at times confusing behaviors of victims of trauma: the seemingly subconscious need to reexperience the traumatic event.

I have treated numerous patients who have been involved in a succession of multiple motor vehicle accidents, in one instance as many as eight MVAs over a twelve-year period. In some cases, these accidents seem to occur with increasing frequency as symptoms of traumatic stress worsen. Some of these accidents may be the result of distractibility due to the effects of trauma and associated dissociation. Others may be related to low-grade hyperarousal, and resulting overreaction to events in traffic. Repeatedly hitting the brakes as a defensive reaction by the hypervigilant driver could well lead to further rear-end collisions. Sometimes the accident is no fault of the victim, and is seemingly inexplicable. One such patient of mine had six rear-end collisions in eighteen months. In many instances, however, traumatic reenactment seems to be driven by more deep-seated unconscious conditioned behavior, and may even be linked to the endorphin-based reward systems noted above.

THE ROOTS OF REENACTMENT

The psychological literature is filled with reports of self-destructive behavior in children and adults with a history of child abuse or with histories of multiple childhood surgeries. Examples include self-mutilation (usually by cutting), self-starvation, and anorexia.[4,5,6] Female victims of childhood physical or sexual abuse have a higher incidence of subsequent abusive male relationships and marriages.[7] Victims of childhood rape or incest are more likely to be raped, and victims of childhood sexual abuse are at higher risk of becoming prostitutes.[8] Some might attribute such behavioral tendencies as being self-destructive or masochistic. It is profoundly inappropriate, however, to pass value judgments on this remarkable association. As you will see, the phenomenon of trauma reenactment is rooted in unconscious biochemical systems of the brain, and is probably a neurophysiologically deep-seated conditioned response.

In a pattern similar to most of the features and behaviors that make up what we call our personality, or self, the roots of trauma reenactment go back to our earliest contacts as an infant with our primary caregiver. Schore explores this maternal/infant interaction in detail.[9] He believes that the earliest verbal, tactile, and auditory interactions between the mother and the infant actually help determine the growth and chemical structure of the brain, leading to the development of personality characteristics and ultimately the person's sense of self. Our basic concepts of the maturation of the individual are dependent on these factors. A healthy, reciprocal maternal interaction provides stability to the arousal systems of the infant brain, and inhibits them from excessive over- or under-responsiveness to threat.[10] The infant deprived of a safe haven in response to his or her caregiver is in an untenable situation. When that caregiver is also a threat, all of the rules are broken, and the child must create his or her own safe reality. Under these circumstances, the child will turn to the only resource available—the abusive caregiver. This is one of the first examples of behavioral constriction, and what we might call inappropriate bonding. The child, however, really has no choice, and will use self-blame to justify reattaching to the abuser, since some sort of attachment or bonding is the child's greatest unconscious need at this age.[11] At times, the child will also resort to provocative behavior, thereby ensuring repetition of the abuse/attachment cycle. This profound, instinctual need for attachment is common to all primate species.[12] Strong evidence supports the fact that this bonding is correlated with heightened levels of endorphins.[13,14] Therefore, attachment bonding by the child is very likely powerfully rewarding even in the face of adrenaline-based arousal caused by bonding with a source of threat, the abusing caregiver.

CLINICAL FEATURES

Endorphins, like other neurotransmitters, clearly serve different functions in different situations. In relation to trauma, they serve to modulate the influence of the traumatic experience, and also to reward the continued bonding that provides infants with the resiliency they require to deal with threat and loss. Thus, children physically abused by their caregiver will experience increased levels of endorphins as part of the traumatization and freeze response. Children will also be rewarded by the presence of increased endorphin levels associated with social reattachment and bonding to the abuser, even in the face of ongoing threat. This same pattern of subjugation, abuse, and passionate reattachment is also typical in many cases of female spousal abuse. It is a fairly accurate reenactment of the similar original child/abusive caregiver bonding. As the conflict leading up to an abusive episode escalates, the abused spouse experiences heightened levels of epinephrine-based arousal, associated with emotions of fear and apprehension. At the same time, release of endorphins provides a subtle sense of familiar pleasure, and even reward.[15] After an episode of abuse, there often is a period of passionate reconciliation accompanied by a further dramatic release of endorphins. This pattern of release of endorphins both with threat and reconciliation provides a powerful reward system for reenactment of the abuse cycle.[16] Analysis of the interaction between couples in an abusive relationship often reveals that the abused member will sometimes trigger abuse with predictable provocative behavior. It is critical in the treatment of spousal abuse to recognize the chemically based features of the relationship to achieve any degree of success. It is also absolutely critical to consider this behavior as being conditioned, not conscious or addictive.

This dual role of brain biochemistry in trauma also probably explains the remarkable phenomenon of the bonding of hostages, kidnap victims, or cult members with their captors.[17] The common feature in these and other abusive situations is the condition of helplessness. The constricting effect of this helplessness cuts the victim off from other sources of support, and like the abused child, the threatened and isolated captive seeks the only source of attachment available, the captor/authority figure.

A fascinating social example of this behavior, one that made the national headlines in the 1970s, is the case of the kidnapping of newspaper heiress Patty Hearst by the radical Symbionese Liberation Army. Within weeks, Ms. Hearst was videotaped by a bank camera, dressed in black combat attire, and wielding an automatic rifle while taking part in a bank robbery with her former captors. In the process, she had developed a sexual/romantic bond with one of the men in the group, and apparently had assumed the group's social identity. The roots of this remarkable and seemingly inexplicable behavior by Ms. Hearst are clearly derived from the same primitive endorphin reward systems of the brain described in abused children and spouses.

Animals show the same stereotyped behavior in the face of threat associated with a state of helplessness. Rats placed in a maze, and given a shock in certain sections of the maze, will typically return compulsively to the threatening area rather than explore safer escape routes. They behave as if the shock and trauma limits their ability to seek out new or different escape options, leading to reenactment of the shock.[18,19] That which is familiar is more rewarding than the unknown even in the face of threat, as in the case of the abused child.

This model of trauma reenactment unfortunately creates a scenario of trauma as a self-fulfilling prophecy. Every time the Vietnam veteran experiences the epinephrine/endorphin arousal/reward response of the combat-related stimulus, that response is reinforced. Every time the abused spouse completes the abuse/reconciliation cycle, it ensures that this cycle will inevitably be repeated between the couple. The brain/biochemistry link in this behavior is quite analogous to the brain biochemistry of narcotic addiction that simply substitutes synthetic morphine derivatives for the brain's natural endorphins.[20] Reenactment therefore constitutes a powerful system of reward and reinforcement, and one that basically is conditioning and self-perpetuating.

GENDER DIFFERENCES

Based on this phenomenon, it is not surprising that persons with childhood trauma, especially when inflicted by their caregiver, are exquisitely sensitive to retraumatization. Studies of trauma victims, however, show remarkable differences between males and females in trauma-related behavior. Males, in general, tend to reenact past trauma by assuming the role of the abusive aggressor rather than that of the victim. As a result, the son of an abusive parent will usually become the abusive spouse or parent as an adult.[21,22] Studies of male criminals convicted of violent aggressive crimes show that a majority of these criminals have suffered severe physical and/or sexual abuse as children.[23,24] These men also appear to have a significantly distorted pain perception consistent with their abnormal brain endorphin systems, and are remarkably prone to various forms of self-mutilation.[6]

Perry studied the posttraumatic behavior patterns of the children released from the Branch Davidian complex in Waco, Texas, after the assault on the complex by agents of the Drug Enforcement Administration in which a number of people were killed.[25] He documented that the male children tended to exhibit anger, aggression, and antisocial behavior. The young girls, however, exhibited anxiety, panic attacks, and sleep disturbance typical of the PTSD symptoms of victimization. He hypothesized that males tend to have an "external locus of control," displacing symptoms of trauma on other members of society, blaming them, and acting out aggressively as a result. Females, however, possess an "internal locus of control," blaming themselves for traumatizing events and manifesting guilt behavior.

This and other examples suggest that female victims of childhood trauma tend to assume the more familiar role of helplessness, and to become attached to and dominated by abusive men. They seem much more sensitive to developing forms of revictimization rather than aggression. Aggressive self-abuse such as self-mutilation is much less common in women than in men. Female victims of abuse or even adult trauma tend to pursue nonviolent, self-destructive activities such as self-starvation. Anorexia nervosa and bulimia are often, if not usually, self-destructive manifestations of trauma reenactment in traumatized young women. The incidence of abuse, especially sexual in nature, is common in women suffering from these conditions.[6]

In natural disaster and accident-related trauma, gender differences may also cause markedly different responses in males and females. Under these conditions, women seem much more likely to experience a more profound freeze, or immobility response, and to sustain that response for a prolonged period. The vast majority of my whiplash patients experiencing prolonged symptoms and delayed recovery have been women. As I have noted, most of my female patients who experienced severe symptoms from trivial auto accidents have a history of significant childhood abuse or medical trauma. The physical and mental symptoms of whiplash can hardly be considered self-rewarding. Nevertheless, the psychic numbing associated with the freeze response and linked to dissociation is clearly a mechanism for pain modulation associated with endorphins, and is therefore rewarding. Adult victims of child abuse have a higher incidence of dissociation in the face of adult trauma. In addition, dissociation, or freezing, at the moment of trauma is associated with a high risk of later development of PTSD (see Chapter 8). These factors probably predispose women to the development of PTSD in traumatic events.

Predictably, men exposed to social trauma, natural disasters, or accidents will respond frequently with rage and aggressive behavior (the fight/flight response), as exemplified by increasingly common "road rage." The degree of violence and aggression seen under these circumstances in men appears to correlate with whether they had experienced abuse and deprivation as children. Admittedly, the victimization/freeze response may also occur in men under these circumstances. This may relate to the complex nature of past traumatic experiences, and to which response, either aggression or freezing, triggers the greatest endorphinergic reward as a result. The roots of gender differences in response to trauma, although probably related in part to theories mentioned, are still not proven. One might speculate that the contribution of genetic influences, relative levels of estrogen and testosterone, or differences in interaction with the maternal caregiver based on gender expectations from the moment of birth could contribute to gender-specific vulnerability. Another disturbing possibility, of course, is the fact that females, both in childhood and as adults, are selectively more exposed to trauma and abuse. Unfortunately, there is a great deal of evidence that this indeed is true as a cross-cultural phenomenon.

Perry and colleagues, however, provide a much more logical and compelling rationale for disparate gender responses to trauma and threat.[25] They base this rationale on the substrate for all brain-related functions, which of course is survival of the species. Using an anthropological and Darwinian model for the behavioral response to threat in males, females, and children, Perry and colleagues address the adaptive advantages of fight, flight, or freeze when facing a life threat in each gender class in members of the primitive tribe or clan. Anthropological literature reflects the tendency in primitive hominid tribes in battle for the victorious tribe to slaughter the adult males of the defeated tribe, and to take the females and children into bondage as property. In the tribe attacked by another tribe, hyperarousal and fighting by children would guarantee death, whereas freezing might allow survival of the children, and their incorporation into the new tribe if their tribe was defeated. The same analogy applies to the tribal female members, whose value in contributing to the victor's gene pool would likely ensure their survival if they also froze. In both cases, the dissociative adaptation to threat by women and children has evolutionary species survival implications. Conversely, if the male members of a threatened tribe were to freeze in the face of this threat, defeat and death would be certain. Sustained hyperarousal in the male tribal members facing threat therefore has great benefit to the survival of the species. Perry and colleagues once again relate this behavioral response to the tendency for males to develop externalized oppositional emotional disorders, and females to develop internalizing disorders such as depression, anxiety, or dissociative disorders.[25]

THE ANNIVERSARY SYNDROME

Another rarely reported but well-documented example of trauma reenactment is what might be called the "anniversary syndrome." Van der Kolk describes a patient who struck a match to light a cigarette while on night patrol in Vietnam in 1968.[26] That brief moment of illumination allowed a Viet Cong sniper to fire at the patrol, and his bullet, in a moment of terrible tragedy, killed the patient's friend. After discharge from the army, the patient found himself apparently unwittingly attempting to rob a store each year, from 1969 to 1986, on the exact day, hour, and minute of the anniversary of the death of his friend. On each occasion, he used his finger in his coat pocket as the "weapon," and waited for the police to arrive, presumably to complete the traumatic experience through his own death.

The similarities between this case history and the actual case from my files at the beginning of this chapter are quite remarkable. How can one explain these seemingly bizarre anniversary-related events in traumatized individuals? One needs to remember that all animals, the human species included, possess innate neurophysiological mechanisms sensitive to the passage of time based on seasonal light variations and even the phases of the moon. The monthly female menstrual cycle may be affected by many subtle outside influences, including the cycles of other females in the household. Subtle seasonal light and temperature characteristics, phases of the moon, or hormonal influences associated with the menstrual cycle at the time of the trauma are very likely stored in implicit memory. Periodic recurrence of these phenomena could result in unconscious activation of arousal on a monthly or even annual basis. Dogs are extremely sensitive to mood changes in their owners. The strange injury described by my patient inflicted by her roommate's pet could be due to secondary arousal of the dog based on subtle biochemical mood changes in my patient related to her past traumatic experience, precipitated by time-contingent internal events. Once again, endorphin-based reward systems associated with this cyclical arousal could well provide further impetus to the repetitive reenactment on the anniversary of the trauma.

REENACTMENT THROUGH RISK TAKING

This strange dance between traumatic arousal and reward also exists in one of our most valued cultural pursuits, high-level athletic competition, especially when involving risk. Although the recent development of the field of extreme sports exemplifies this phenomenon, it exists at many levels and is probably proportionate to the level of intrinsic effort or risk of the particular event. Thus, the release of epinephrine in the face of threat to survival may be associated not only with feelings of anxiety and fear, but also with excitement and exhilaration. One might easily speculate that this disparity could be explained by the relative balance of epinephrine and endorphin release with the specific experience.

A person's first skydiving parachute jump is typically associated with stomach-churning panic. Thereafter, the exhilaration and "high" tends to replace fear and trepidation with eager anticipation. That "high" is so great in extreme sports that participants will often pursue the event with a degree of intensity consistent with addictive behavior. Examples of this kind of extreme sport include free jumping (off of buildings, towers, or cliffs), extreme skiing, boating or driving to set speed records, technical rock climbing without ropes, and high altitude mountaineering. All of these sports involve a potentially life-threatening pursuit with superficially intangible rewards. All are associated with initial fear, followed by exhilaration and reward, followed by compulsive pursuit of the activity. Often this risk-taking behavior is associated with "upping the ante," by increasing the difficulty and danger of the pursuit in order to increase the reward.

All such dangerous pursuits are connected with a powerful fear-based arousal, without which the process will not be initiated. Once established, the fear response no longer seems necessary to perpetuate the habitual thrill response. In every sense of the definition, this thrill-seeking behavior is analogous to more destructive traumatic reenactment. It is governed by the same adrenaline/endorphin threat/reward systems that characterize the behavior of the abused spouse. Although clearly less dramatic, the endorphin withdrawal between episodes of exhilaration has many of the characteristics of morphine withdrawal: restlessness, anxiety, disturbance of sleep, and preoccupation with reproducing the activity.[17]

Those sports that involve maximal sustained physical exertion and effort and that are associated with the most severe anaerobic pain probably are also closely linked to the cycle of traumatic arousal and reward characteristics of reenactment. The "runner's high" has been described at length since the boom in recreational running began in the 1970s. This "high" has been linked to the release of endorphins triggered by this unique physical activity, and this relationship between exertion and endorphin release has been reasonably well validated. Marathons, ultramarathons, triathlons, and competitive cycling are all associated with intense aerobic and anaerobic pain and are probably rewarded and facilitated by endorphin release. In these instances, the stimulus appears to be pain rather than fear. Without this pain, the ultimate reward is substantially lessened.

The necessary practice of intense training to reach sufficient fitness levels to achieve a reasonable level of competition in these sports is by definition painful, at times agonizingly so. Athletes in these circumstances comment on the pain, but often refer to the experience as being "in the zone," a condition of distraction that almost certainly has its roots in the endorphin-based condition of dissociation. The time commitment involved often precludes a meaningful social or even family life outside of the training and competition.

This feature of endurance training is probably true to a much greater extent than in typical seasonal game-based sports. In addition, the financial rewards outside of the core of elite athletes in endurance sports are negligible. Yet even those athletes at the fringe of competition, with no hope of victory, wealth, or recognition, continue to pursue the same painful, self-sacrificing lifestyle, driven presumably by the same mechanisms of endorphin reward that characterize trauma reenactment.

In conversations with trainers and physicians who treat elite endurance athletes, I find a kernel of evidence that this pursuit of fear or pain-based arousal and reward is related at times to a history of childhood trauma or abuse. This presumption is admittedly speculative at best. But it makes sense, and is consistent with the basic principles of trauma reenactment, that victims of childhood trauma would find the endorphin-based rewards of endurance and extreme sports very powerful. If this association is indeed valid, intense athletic pursuit represents a relatively healthy and stable means of managing the powerful forces driving the victim of trauma toward reenactment. Unfortunately, the serious injury and fatality rate in some of these sports raises questions about implications for species survival.

In less extreme risk-taking athletic pursuits, the same reward system certainly exists. The thrill of competition, especially when victorious, is a powerful narcotic, as any athlete will agree. Clearly it is not the financial reward that makes players compete well beyond their prime, even when permanent physical impairment may result. The boxer who returns to the ring in his forties and the football quarterback who continues to play despite painful, damaged knees are spurred on by the endorphin-based rewards of "the game." Endorphins serve an important phylogenetic role in allowing wounded prey animals to escape the predator by inhibiting the need to minister to their wounds. The same phenomenon may also drive the human creature to continue to pursue this endorphinergic reward at the risk of health and survival.

CONCLUSION

In a sense, our species' survival may be dependent on these conditioned mechanisms whereby we push on beyond fear and pain to achieve a goal. Endorphin-based reward systems have evolved as a means of facilitating behavior that is specific to survival, not as a means of perpetuating reenactment. If the neurochemical changes of traumatic stress have resulted from dissociation and a truncated freeze response, however, the result may be endorphinergic reward for reenactment rather than survival. Once again the phenomenon of dissociation may serve as the fuel for another of the features of PTSD. Within this context, however, may lie other neurochemical forces that drive gender-based behavioral responses to traumatic stress. Just as changes in brain chemistry and function associated with the experience of trauma may lead to specific diseases of the body, they may also lead to inexplicable behavioral changes such as trauma reenactment. These late effects of traumatic stress reflect the complexity of the process, and suggest that there may be many pathways to behavioral dysfunction resulting from trauma that merit exploration well beyond the defined concept of PTSD.

Chapter 8

Somatic Dissociation

Sam had suffered fractures of his right wrist and ankle in a particularly traumatic head-on motor vehicle accident. Thereafter, along with significant PTSD, he developed intractable burning pain, associated with variable heat and coolness of the right hand and foot. This condition was eventually diagnosed as reflex sympathetic dystrophy (RSD), a particularly malignant and painful condition that occasionally follows injuries. Despite extensive treatment including multiple sympathetic blocks, treatment in a pain center, and multiple medication trials, Sam was ultimately disabled by his RSD. His physical examination revealed measurable increased warmth along the outside of his right lower leg and foot, and coolness of his right hand, with extreme painful sensitivity to touch of the skin in those areas. I performed visual boundary testing during one of his visits with me. As I held my outstretched hand in the range of his right visual field at a distance of about four feet, he flushed and experienced discomfort. When I asked him what he had experienced, he told me that he had felt a flash of anger toward me. He then had a sudden memory of his grandfather striking him on the back of his right leg with a fireplace poker as a child, a preferred form of punishment in his family. His RSD had developed in an injured leg that was incorporated in a region of his perceptual field that held a persistent latent threat to his sense of safety. This was the region of his body that had experienced repeated, painful traumatic messages as a child.

* * *

Dissociation is a term coined by Janet in the late nineteenth century to describe mental states in which a disruption of conscious awareness occurs.[1] In this state of altered consciousness, the individual may experience distortion of memory, affect, perception, or sense of identity. The affected person may experience altered perceptions of somatic sensations and time, periods of amnesia, unreality, and depersonalization. More profound clinical states include conversion symptoms, fugue states, and multiple personality disorder (dissociative identity disorder).[2-5] Psychiatrists believed that dissociation occurred when anxiety became so overwhelming that certain aspects of the personality became dissociated or split from one another. They believed that the various manifestations of dissociation served to protect the individual from the conflict producing the anxiety. Dissociation, in other words, served as a psychological escape mechanism from fear.

EXAMPLES OF DISSOCIATION

In the traumatized person, dissociation occurs in many forms, at many times in the evolution of traumatic stress and post-traumatic stress disorder, and has emotional, perceptual, physical, and memory-related manifestations. In a motor vehicle accident, dissociation presents as the emotional and perceptual confusion and numbness often experienced at the time of the accident. The freeze or immobility response itself very likely represents a type, or perhaps a part, of dissociation. The out-of-body, third-person perception that people sometimes feel at the moment of traumatic stress is an example of *depersonalization,* a classic symptom of dissociation. The victim of childhood incest who perceives her disembodied self as looking down from the ceiling of her bedroom feeling sorry for the little girl on the bed being abused by her father is experiencing this form of dissociation.

Several of my MVA patients have described this phenomenon vividly. One patient was sitting in the front passenger seat of a car driven by a friend. They stopped at his mountain home after a trip as they completed a conversation. Suddenly, she saw from her left a car traveling erratically down the steep road toward them. As the car lost control and hurtled over an embankment toward their car, she began to perceive events as occurring in slow motion, and then realized that she was looking down on the scene from above the car, in which she could still see herself sitting next to the driver. The oncoming car then descended through the air, landed on the hood of their car, bounced off, and landed on its top ten feet from their car. During this shocking event, the patient remained calm and detached. She then found herself "back in her body," unhurt and apparently unshaken. She calmly exited the car and went to check on the driver's son, who had climbed out of the car before the impact to check the mail. She then checked on the driver of the other car, and went into the house to call the police and ambulance. All of this was done in apparent complete emotional control, although later she would report that she did all of this in a state of "automatic pilot." The next morning she awoke with an agonizing headache and neck pain, and thereafter experienced the full- blown whiplash syndrome that I have described, even though the car in which she was sitting was shaken but not moved by the impact. Her symptoms included intractable headache and neck pain, prominent cognitive impairment, and full-blown acute PTSD.

Another patient involved in a moderate impact, rear-end MVA experienced a profound out-of-body experience similar to the one described previously. When she emerged from her car, she experienced a sudden revelation that the heavens opened up and filled her with an amazing power with the implication that it would forever change her life. She even perceived a bright light in the sky at the time. This is called *derealization,* the sense that immediate perceptions are unreal, or in this case supernatural, and is another example of dissociation.[4] Not surprisingly, an experience such as the one just described might be considered delusional, and in this case the doctors who evaluated the patient in the emergency room believed that she was probably a psychiatric patient.

Almost all of my patients with clinical PTSD after an MVA say that they have lost their sense of self, that they no longer know who they are, and that they are now living a strange and unrecognizable life. This sense of unreality pervades their life, and is often referred to as a "fog" that exists between them and their sense of awareness and the rest of the world. Although this foglike perception is often described as almost palpable, its main feature seems to be a clouding of consciousness, both cognitive and emotional, with numbing, distraction, and loss of emotional tone. At times in the course of a patient's recovery, this "fog" may lift rather suddenly, and this event is almost always associated with improvement in cognitive impairment. Symptoms of arousal and hypervigilence actually may increase with clearing of this state of numbing. Dissociative symptoms in general are indeed often bizarre by the usual medical standards and often seem to defy rational physical explanation. In my experience, however, the clearing of this sense of clouded perception is frequently a positive result of therapy for the trauma.

Perhaps the most extreme instance of depersonalization in dissociation involves the development of multiple personality, or dissociative identity disorder. This rare condition is clearly an example of traumatic dissociation, with the incidence of severe child abuse in these individuals approaching 80 percent.[6] The various personalities exhibited in this disorder may show difference in hand and apparent cerebral hemispheric dominance, different psychophysiological responses to stress, and may even suffer from different diseases as evidence for remarkable physiological and somatic dissociation.

MEMORY IN DISSOCIATION

Distortions of memory in PTSD may also be a manifestation of dissociation. Traumatic amnesia is perhaps the most common example.[7] Whereas many traumatized patients experience recurring and intrusive memories of the trauma, a significant number have partial or complete amnesia for the experience. This form of amnesia is especially common in adult survivors of child abuse, who may have little if any memory for their abuse,[8] or remember it in grossly distorted terms. Although recovered memories of child abuse may be distorted or inaccurate, they often do indeed represent dissociative amnesia for actual events.

Many victims of child abuse may have remarkably little memory for *any* events of their childhood as a result of this process. Several of my MVA victims, suffering from amnesia for an accident presumed to be due to a head injury, have recovered complete memory for details of the accident with trauma therapy alone. Memories for the traumatic event may also be distorted by the perceptual alterations associated with a traumatic experience.[9] The process of derealization leads to remarkable memory alterations, including the clear memory of an out-of-body experience.[4] The memory for the sense of the passage of time is often greatly altered,[10] and usually is experienced as the dramatic slowing of time, "as if my life passed before my eyes." Frequently sounds, smells, and other sensations are greatly amplified in traumatic memory as part of the dissociative experience. In MVAs, the impact is often described as "a bomb going off." The powder released by the air bag is remembered as "suffocating." As the traumatized individual cycles in and out of dissociation, these somatic memories may serve as conditioned cues that may trigger panic, flashbacks, and somatic dissociative symptoms.

The most profound type of dissociative amnesia is called a fugue state. In its most dramatic form, this type of dissociation is probably what the Hollywood movie industry is trying to represent in fictional stories about persons suffering prolonged periods of amnesia. These persons are depicted as suffering profound emotional trauma, or sometimes a blow to the head. Thereafter, the victims go so far as to begin another life with no memory for prior life events, including their own name or past life history. Although obviously stretching reality in the interests of drama, these stories have a kernel of truth.

A fugue state is often characterized by a prolonged time for which the patients have no memory, but during which they continue to talk and relate in a somewhat normal fashion. During this time, they may not remember their name or personal facts, but otherwise appear normal. In other fugue states, they may appear confused, dramatic or histrionic, socially inappropriate, or bizarre. When such a fugue state clears, as it eventually does, the patients usually have no memory of the events that occurred during that time. This type of reaction occurring in the context of an MVA usually occurs at the time of, or just after, the accident. Once again this may be difficult to distinguish from the occasionally confused behavior that may accompany a closed head injury. During the amnestic period following a moderate closed head injury, agitated, delusional, or even combative behavior may occur that later may be very difficult to distinguish from similar behavior due to a traumatically induced fugue state.

Another dissociative memory disturbance, also seen in a number of my whiplash patients, is the loss of memory for remote, familiar events, some of them containing strong personal emotional content. Although this phenomenon is often attributed to the effects of a minor traumatic brain injury, these patients have accurate recall of the accident itself, and in addition to cognitive complaints, all of them had other dissociative and arousal symptoms of PTSD. Selective amnesia for remote events in these patients is very likely dissociative in nature, and relates to similar traumatic amnesia for childhood events in victims of child abuse.

Actual flashback memories associated with trauma also represent dissociative events. They are almost always associated with intense emotional arousal, and often panic.[11] During a flashback memory, the patient's sense of awareness and reality is usually distorted, with a sense of detachment from one's immediate surroundings. The patient may report the "foglike" sense previously described, and other sensations may be similarly altered. Memory associated with the flashback will almost always relate to the specific trauma and may be quite accurate, but also may be altered, exaggerated, symbolic, or otherwise distorted from the actual event. Flashbacks may last from minutes to hours, or even days. Needless to say, the person is essentially completely disabled during the flashback experience, both from the confusion accompanying the memory and the associated intense arousal. Flashbacks as well as repeated intrusive memories of a traumatic event are representative of the fact that memory in trauma, in addition to being absent for certain events, may also be exaggerated and excessive. Unlike the dissociative nature of flashbacks, intrusive memories tend to be more accurate and representative of the traumatic experience, perhaps even more so than common declarative memories unlinked to emotion or arousal.[12]

COGNITIVE AND EMOTIONAL FEATURES

Dissociative symptoms in trauma also affect attention, cognition, and emotional intensity, mainly by constriction, withdrawal, and detachment. All of these behaviors serve to protect traumatized persons from experiencing arousal by literally removing them from the scene of the action. Constriction impairs both the victim's awareness of events around them and the emotions associated with those events. Mood, affect, and range of emotion may be blunted and flattened. Fear and panic may be dulled, but joy, pleasure, and satisfaction may be muted as well. Social isolation may accompany withdrawal, and may become so complete that the trauma victim may literally become a hermit. The image of the traumatized Vietnam veteran retreating to a cabin in the forest, as depicted in several motion pictures, is not entirely exaggerated.

Detachment may produce a distorted sense of time. The victims may spend their days in random and disjointed behavior, missing meals, not attending to personal hygiene, and confusing night and day. Neglect and confusion of purpose may be severe and quite disabling. Conversely, trauma victims may rigidly plan every hour of their waking day in order to avoid the intrusion of anxiety that appears whenever they do not have everything in their life scheduled, planned, and organized. Obsessive-compulsive behaviors may result from this aspect of traumatic stress. Such patients will organize and reorganize details of their life, especially as they relate to the MVA after whiplash. They may drive the medical provider to distraction with constant requests and demands to deal with what they perceive to be daily life crises, with many of these demands being perseverative and anxiety-driven. These patients are very likely to review the copy of the medical consult that the physician has performed, and to make multiple minute corrections of facts as related to the case history described in that report.

Other problems of cognitive and mental processing functions may result from dissociation. Constricted attention may affect the person's ability to access information, with distraction leading the person to neglect and ignore the details of the information that is heard, seen, or read. This symptom may often present as forgetfulness, absent-mindedness, or simply as an attention deficit. In fact, in PTSD patients, neuropsychological test batteries reveal a variety of deficits, usually in the areas of short-term memory and attention.[13-19] Adult victims of trauma have more recently been diagnosed as having adult ADD (attention deficit disorder). They may also show impaired higher-level intellectual information processing and executive function. The ability to make judgments based on complex pieces of information and the ability to problem solve based on complex associations may be dulled.[20,21] They may neglect the details in making decisions, instead reaching conclusions based mainly on initially constricted impressions. This process of constriction may limit access to the full range of available information and, as a result, common sense, judgment, and logic may at times be impaired, or stereotyped. Often the victims of trauma, sensing the difficulties associated with cognitive demands, may make every effort to avoid participating in life decisions in order to reduce the complexity of their life.

The literature cited previously documents significant cognitive impairment in trauma survivors unexplained by coincidental minor brain injury. I have noted in many of my whiplash trauma victims that test scores on neuropsychological test batteries are even worse than one would expect from their apparent level of daily function. Several such patients have completed college and graduate level degrees with neuropsychological test scores that would suggest that this achievement should not be feasible. I believe that the very process of exposure to the demands of this type of testing may accentuate fear and anxiety, trigger distraction and dissociation, and lead to artificially depressed test scores.

DISSOCIATIVE PHYSICAL SYMPTOMS

Perhaps the least appreciated manifestations of dissociation in trauma are in the areas of perceptual alterations and somatic symptoms. As noted, time perception is often altered, especially with the dissociative response associated with the initial traumatic freeze episode.[11] The popularly described sensation of "time standing still" is indeed a frequent perception of the MVA victim at the moment of impact, as documented in hundreds of my patients. Slowing of time is the most common alteration of time perception. A sense of time alteration may persist for some time after the impact, and its duration often reflects the length of time of the post-MVA freeze episode, or period of dissociation.

Visual perception and acuity are also commonly affected in dissociation. Flashback memories are often characterized by marked distortion of shape and color, usually with vivid and bizarre changes that reflect the accompanying state of enhanced arousal, as noted in prior references to MVA experiences. The MVA victim will often remember the other car in flashbacks and intrusive memories as being enlarged and distorted, and traveling at exaggerated speeds. In earlier chapters, we discussed the frequent association of binocular visual acuity impairment and convergence insufficiency in whiplash patients. These patients often also have less easily explained monocular visual alteration, including monocular diplopia and blurring of vision in one eye.

One such patient was referred to me because of partial vision loss in her right eye following an auto accident two months prior. She had not experienced a blow to her head. The patient had lost control of her car on an icy mountain road, and as the car spun out of control, it slid off of the right side of the road into a shallow ditch. On the other side of the ditch was a cliff. As she watched the edge of the cliff approaching from her right side (perceived in slow motion of course), her car was stopped by impacting a tree, and came to rest. Thereafter, she developed persistent blurring of vision in her right eye. Ocular refraction showed a consistent refractive error that appeared to be correctable, and she was fitted with a lens that provided clear vision in that eye. Within minutes after putting on the glasses with the new lens, she developed nausea, palpitations, flashback memories of the accident, and panic. Any further attempts to restore or correct the measurable refractive error in her right eye continued to produce attacks of panic and reexperiencing of the traumatic event through flashbacks. Her visual impairment was diagnosed as being hysterical in nature.

This remarkable patient presents an example of this group of symptoms. The measurable but physically unexplained refractive error in her right eye was clearly a somatic dissociative response driven by the moment of life-threatening danger perceived in that eye at the time of the MVA. Visual images perceived in her right eye activated procedural memory for the terrifying events of the potentially fatal accident and triggered emotionally valenced flashbacks and panic. Blurring of vision in that eye became a protective dissociative phenomenon. The unusual feature of this case, of course, is that the refractive error was consistently measurable and reproducible. Dissociation had resulted in a probably temporary but physiologically measurable alteration in the dissociated end organ. The occurrence of this type of visual distortion in MVAs usually appears related to the association of visual cues accompanying the threat at the moment of the accident. In my patient population, it occurs much less often in rear-end accidents in which the victim did not see the car approaching, and is especially common when direct visual input of the impending threat occurred from one side or the other.

Distortion of proprioceptive awareness of the victim's body is a common dissociative phenomenon. This is often associated with an injured part or region of the body, especially one of the extremities. The patient will note altered sensation, usually a vague sense of numbness, but the exact sensation is usually very difficult to describe. The extremity may be neglected or ignored, and postural abnormalities may result that can be quite remarkable. Examination of the part of the body involved may reveal sensory changes on a variety of tests that will usually be interpreted as "nonphysiological" in nature by the physician. Stocking or glove patterns of loss of pain, touch, and vibratory sensation are common. Strength testing often shows giveaway weakness.

Patients presenting with these neurological findings will frequently be diagnosed as suffering from conversion hysteria.

A remarkable example of somatic dissociation was seen in an MVA victim treated in my chronic pain program. This young lady had been involved in a rollover accident during which her left arm was crushed by the car as it rolled, tearing off almost the entire skin of her forearm. Amazingly, she suffered minimal nerve damage, but required extensive skin grafting of the forearm. The sensation in the grafted skin was obviously deadened and never returned to normal, but as she recovered she developed increasing vague, hard to describe aching pain that was resistant to all treatment, although it did not fulfill criteria for sympathetically maintained pain. She essentially stopped using the arm and hand for any activity. The pain was actually worse in the shoulder than the forearm, and was associated with some evidence of myofascial pain and spasm in the shoulder. The remarkable feature of her physical examination, however, was her posture. In the standing position, her head was side bent and rotated to the right, and her torso was also rotated to the right. Her left shoulder blade was rotated backward and the arm almost held behind her, literally out of her view. She was totally unaware of this position of total rejection and dissociation of her entire left arm, even when looking in a mirror. When shown a face-on, full-body photograph of herself, however, she was surprised and shocked at her unusual appearance. With trauma therapy and postural education, the pain largely disappeared in a sequential fashion as her posture approached a more normal status.

In our chronic pain program, we invariably see that the patients' unconscious posture reflects not only their pain, but also the experience of the traumatic event that produced the pain. The asymmetrical postural patterns, held in procedural memory, almost always reflect the body's attempt to move away from the injury or threat that caused the injury. Many of these patients manifest the "nonphysiological findings" that have branded them as chronic pain patients by their physicians. With careful exploration of the mechanisms of the source of the pain, however, one will usually find strong evidence for a history of traumatic stress specific to that area of the body. Specific neuromuscular postural patterns that have developed related to their injury are often visible markers for the presence of somatic dissociation, and explain the patterns of "nonphysiological findings."

CONVERSION AND DISSOCIATION

Even nonpsychiatric physicians generally place nonphysiological findings in the diagnostic category of a "conversion reaction," or conversion hysteria. This psychiatric condition was described in detail by Janet and Freud.[1,2] As noted earlier, conversion is considered to be a protection against intolerable levels of anxiety or phobias. The anxiety is "converted" into symptoms in organs or other parts of the body, and usually presents as sensory or motor neurological symptoms. These symptoms tend to represent the mental conflict creating the anxiety, and also meet some need of the patient—provide "secondary gain"—on an unconscious basis. Conversion of an intolerable anxiety to a physical symptom indeed provides great emotional relief, hence the frequently documented indifference to the disabling physical condition *(la belle indifference)*. Hysterical paralysis, for example, has been seen regularly in traumatized soldiers suffering from "shell shock" or "battle fatigue." Hysterical paraplegia at the turn of the century was classically attributed in women to sexual ambivalence—i.e., to a confused mixture of erotic feelings and disgust with regard to sexuality.[2] The very term "hysteria" derives from the Greek word for the uterus, *hystera*, essentially branding conversion reaction as a feminine condition. These young women were initially suspected, and are now thought to have been, victims of incest, and the secondary gain achieved is now believed to have been a form of protection from further exposure to their source of trauma.

In the DSM-IV, conversion has been assigned to the category of somatiform disorders, and is technically not felt to represent a true dissociative disorder. As part of the thesis of this chapter, however, I believe that all somatiform disorders constitute subsets of the dissociative response, and that they have a measurable physiological basis and origin. Conversion reaction, then, is an example of regional somatic dissociation as a reaction to trauma.

It is apparent that the patient with a conversion reaction will almost always have been a victim of trauma in the past, usually in addition to the new trauma that may have precipitated the conversion symptoms. Often this past trauma will have been severe childhood abuse. Children typically dissociate in the face of traumatic stress, as we have noted. They sustain this tendency to freeze in the face of perceived threat as they grow older, with each episode of dissociation tending to reinforce the susceptibility to freeze in the face of subsequent threat. As a result, adults with a history of child abuse typically experience a greater tendency to freeze at the moment of subsequent trauma and to develop dissociative symptoms. Dissociation is the primary predictor for the later development of PTSD.[22] Individuals who actively dissociate at the time of a traumatic event are much more likely to develop subsequent symptoms of PTSD than those who do not.[23-25] People with a history of trauma or PTSD also are susceptible to arousal, freezing, and retraumatization after exposure to arousal stimuli unrelated to prior traumatic life experiences.[26] They also have trouble differentiating relevant from irrelevant stimuli with regard to content and meaning of threat.[27] The tendency to freeze in the face of trauma appears to be a self-fulfilling prophecy, rendering the victim increasingly sensitive to traumatization with ever-decreasing severity and specificity of threat exposure. This phenomenon of sensitization to increasingly minor and apparently irrelevant threat in victims of childhood trauma, may well explain the remarkable incidence of dissociative symptoms and PTSD in my patients with a history of childhood trauma injured in relatively trivial MVAs.

Although poorly understood, a number of neurophysiological processes likely contribute to the clinical phenomenon of dissociation. Recently, attention has been drawn to the role of the dorsal medial prefrontal cortex (MPFC), or anterior cingulate, in PTSD.[28] Reference has been made to this region with regard to concepts of brain plasticity in PTSD in Chapter 5. Hamner noted that lesions of the anterior cingulate may facilitate the acquisition of fear conditioning, suggesting that this region may provide a gating function inhibiting fear conditioning.[29] You will recall that the amygdala receives input from the locus ceruleus in states of potential threat, and evaluates that information for its emotional or arousal-based content. Continued activation of the amygdala by further input from the locus ceruleus may then set up a state of fear conditioning. The gating or control function of the anterior cingulate is believed to occur through inhibition of activation of the amygdala at the time of fear arousal. Lack of this inhibition of fear conditioning by the cingulate may lead to increased sensitivity to internal and external trauma-related cues.

In Hamner's model, inhibition of the anterior cingulate by excessive adrenergic input from the locus ceruleus with traumatic arousal may limit this gating function of the cingulate on the amygdala. This in turn, would allow exposure of the amygdala to overwhelming internal and external arousal cues, thereby producing the exaggerated emotional and behavioral symptoms of PTSD. Once established, locus ceruleus/amygdala kindling would continue to suppress anterior cingulate function, and perpetuate the conditioned fear response (see Figure 8.1). In addition, the anterior cingulate appears to play a role in emotionality, selective attention, and certain social functions, including emotional attachments and parenting, as well as generation of the concept of the self in relation to society. Fragmentation of these functions through inhibition of the anterior cingulate in PTSD may explain the inability of its victims to form social bonds, to manifest avoidance and isolation, and to experience fragmentation of the sense of self that typifies dissociation.

Dissociation almost certainly is also mediated at least in part by endorphinergic influences, which may in turn explain the dissociative phenomena of numbing, confusion, and cognitive impairment. Certainly the analgesia associated with the freeze, or immobility, response— the precursor and extreme expression of dissociation—is related to endorphinergic mediation. Current theory also strongly relates endogenous opioids to the phenomenon of trauma reenactment.[30] Increasing sensitization to dissociate in the face of threat may well be based on opioid reward systems.

Dissociation, or freezing, may represent the perpetuating mechanism that fuels the kindled arousal/memory feedback circuit of sustained PTSD. If so, it may be the reason why victims of prior traumatic stress, especially childhood abuse, are so susceptible to the development of PTSD symptoms in otherwise minor episodes of life stress, including low velocity MVAs, as noted in my patient population. The underlying neurochemistry and neurophysiology of dissociation is likely to be of critical importance to the understanding of its role in trauma.

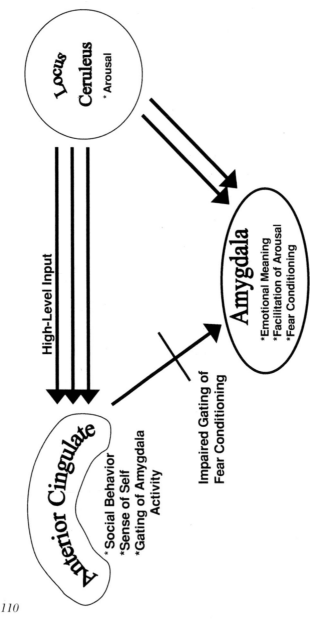

FIGURE 8.1. Theoretical role of the anterior cingulate in post-traumatic stress disorder. The anterior cingulate may exert a braking action on activation of the amygdala, and therefore provide a gating mechanism on the development of fear conditioning in traumatic stress. Excessive or prolonged arousal input from the locus ceruleus in unresolved trauma may impair this gating action through cingulate inhibition, thereby potentiating fear conditioning and traumatic kindling in PTSD.

THE AUTONOMIC NERVOUS SYSTEM
IN POST-TRAUMATIC STRESS DISORDER

Dissociation may also result in, or conversely be a manifestation of, the splitting of symptoms related to exaggerated cyclical tone of the autonomic nervous system. Many of my patients, during the early stages after an MVA, when they are still in the numb and stunned phase of the freeze response, complain of recurrent diarrhea and abdominal cramps, nausea, and indigestion.

A remarkable young woman with preceding obsessive-compulsive disorder suffered soft tissue injuries in a relatively high-speed rear-end accident in which her car was totally destroyed. Following the accident, she had mild neck pain and headache easily controlled with over-the-counter analgesics, but no other elements of the whiplash syndrome. She was remarkably free from symptoms of arousal and of PTSD, and had no cognitive or emotional complaints, although her preexisting reclusive behavior patterns were accentuated. Within two weeks, however, she developed persistent and disabling watery diarrhea. Extensive gastrointestinal investigation by a gastroenterologist, including multiple stool cultures, failed to reveal any pathological cause for the diarrhea, which lasted for several months. With the initiation of a somatic behavioral trauma therapy directed at trauma resolution, she began to have normal bowel movements. As the diarrhea subsided, however, she began to experience the emergence of symptoms of arousal, including anxiety attacks, driving phobias, nightmares, and cognitive symptoms.

It is apparent that the process of her dissociation was initially associated with dramatic parasympathetic activation, with relative suppression of sympathetic arousal. Partial resolution of her dissociation through therapy unfortunately, but probably predictably, resulted in appearance of arousal symptoms consistent with PTSD. Any form of psychotherapy has the risk of flooding or releasing arousal in the dissociated patient. In this case, return to a more sympathetically dominant state resulted in temporary clearing of severe parasympathetic somatic symptoms, suggesting the role of parasympathetic dominance in dissociation.

This role of the autonomic nervous system in the perpetuation of the arousal/dissociation cycle of PTSD is of particular importance to this discussion. Criteria for the diagnosis of PTSD in the DSM-IV do not specifically refer to it as a cyclical disease, but the bipolar extremes of the symptoms addressed (extreme arousal ↔ extreme avoidance) lend themselves to this consideration.[31] The three criteria categories of PTSD in the DSM-IV (reexperiencing, avoidance, and arousal) reflect dramatic swings of mood, ranging from panic, hypervigilence, and irritability to numbing, detachment, and flattened affect. Physiological markers for PTSD referenced in the DSM-IV include measurements of pulse rate, and electromyographic and electrodermal responses, all primarily measurements of sympathetic autonomic activity. The role of parasympathetic activation or tone in PTSD, however, has been largely neglected.

Oscillatory phenomena in neurophysiological and behavioral systems have been documented in a variety of settings. Antelman and colleagues propose that the exposure of such systems (e.g., endocrine, autonomic, neurohumoral) to chemical or behavioral stressors can induce cyclical patterns of increase and decrease in response to each subsequent exposure.[32-34] This phenomenon occurs in such a diversity of systems that oscillation in response to chemical or behavioral input may well represent a general principle of biological functioning.[35] Exposure of such systems to stressors sufficient to produce oscillation is entirely analogous to the theories of sensitization and kindling in PTSD (see Chapter 4). A system, such as the autonomic nervous system, sensitized by exposure to stressors without physiological resolution of the resulting response, will be driven to reverberate, or oscillate, within the limits of its physiological boundaries. This may well be an innate biological reflex designed to reestablish homeostasis, the rhythmic and balanced subtle fluctuation of all body systems, be they endocrinologic, neurophysiologic, metabolic, or immunologic.[35] If this sensitized system continues to be bombarded by stressors, homeostasis will be prevented, and the exaggerated oscillatory cycles will continue. In the case of PTSD, internal kindled neurophysiological circuits perpetuated by the lack of resolution of a conditioned fight/flight response may provide internal sensitized arousal-based stressors that serve to perpetuate autonomic oscillation. The result is a perpetuated and excessive cyclical dysfunction of autonomic regulation leading to the alternating symptom categories of arousal and avoidance in the traumatized individual (see Figure 8.2). Exaggerated autonomic oscillation also explains the bipolar somatic manifestations of MVA victims with PTSD, ranging from sympathetic activation of neuromuscular

protective responses (muscle bracing, bruxism) to vegetative gastro-intestinal symptoms (acid reflux, abdominal cramps, diarrhea). Since hyperarousal is also known to be associated with increased release of endogenous opioids, internal reward systems may well contribute to the perpetuation of this exaggerated autonomic cycling.

If you will recall, in Chapter 5 we reviewed findings of depressed levels of serum cortisol in those patients with chronic PTSD. Associated with this unusual finding is evidence for a sensitized hypothalamic/pituitary/adrenal axis in these patients in that they respond to a dexamethasone suppression test with *exaggerated* suppression of serum cortisol levels. In the normal response to threat, serum cortisol is elevated by stress and arousal through HPA activation and in turn inhibits continued activation of the HPA axis, thus modulating the brain's acute response to stress. Continued and repetitive stress exposure would be expected to result in sustained elevation of serum cortisol. In PTSD, however, the "stress" to which the patient is subjected is internal, through kindled memory systems that are activated by spontaneous recycled memories, and also activated by increasingly nonspecific external stress-linked cues. Since these types of stressors are not amenable to resistance or escape, the inevitable response is a cyclical and increasingly recurrent freeze, or dissociative response. Dissociation is a state of marked parasympathetic activation, one that is associated with reduced muscular and cardiovascular tone. In chronic PTSD, avoidance symptoms become increasingly prominent, as manifested by progressive social isolation, substance abuse, and constricted affect.

Avoidance, denial, and dissociation share many clinical and psychophysiological features, and in general reflect parasympathetic dominance. Depressed serum cortisol in PTSD therefore may well be a reflection of late prominence of parasympathetic influences on its chronic state. On the other hand, there is evidence that the HPA axis in PTSD may be more sensitive and in fact overresponsive to internal biological stimuli. This may reflect neurophysiological sensitization and kindling phenomena also attributed to trauma.[36] This finding is also in keeping with the cyclical model of autonomic fluctuation in PTSD. In late PTSD, however, the cycle is spent increasingly in the parasympathetically dominant states of depression, dissociation, and somatization, as avoidance increasingly isolates the patient from arousal-based cues.

The most compelling model for the evolution of the parasympathetic response to stress lies in the study of infant brain maturation based on early social experience. In his review of the pediatric developmental psychobiological literature, Schore discusses the evolving state of infant brain development on the basis of reactive autonomic oscillation.[37] In the dyadic emotional interaction between mother and child, a negative maternal response will elicit a state of shame/withdrawal, characterized by a shift from sympathetic "ergotrophic" arousal, to parasympathetic "trophotrophic" arousal, from a hyperaroused to a hypoaroused state. Parasympathetic neurohumoral responses will accompany this shift, including decreased muscle tone, withdrawal from social interaction, vasodilatation (blushing), and loss of facial expression. This phenomenon has been called "conservation withdrawal," and clearly represents the early manifestation of the freeze or dissociative response in trauma. Although the development of socialized behavior patterns seems dependent on this process, a pattern of excessive elicitation of this shame response will result in inadequate development of coping strategies by the infant, and contribute to the development of psychiatric and characterologic disturbances.[37]

Schore believes that maturational development of the right orbitofrontal cortex (OFC), the primary regulator of autonomic stability, may actually be inhibited by excessive elicitation of shame, rendering these infants more vulnerable to withdrawal. Impaired development of this cortical area through impaired dyadic maternal attunement clearly would render the child and later the adult more vulnerable to the unstable and abnormal oscillatory autonomic state described above, and render the individual more vulnerable to traumatization by stressors of relatively less severity. Impaired physiological and anatomical development of the right OFC may therefore represent the most critical factor in the vulnerability of neglected or traumatized infants or children to later traumatic life events.

Further insights regarding the phylogenetic role of the parasympathetic nervous system in PTSD may be drawn from specifics of the Polyvagal Theory of Emotion as presented by Porges.[38] These insights amplify the importance of sustained parasympathetic tone in dissociation and the perpetuation of the syndrome. Porges emphasizes the phylogenetic layering of arousal responses in mammals, based on the varied functions of the vagal nuclei. The dorsal vagal complex (DVC), composed of the dorsal motor nucleus of the vagus and nucleus tractus solitarius, is a vestigial and primitive center, primarily useful in reptiles for energy conservation. In the low oxygen-demand system of the reptile, the DVC shuts down the energy-use system by inducing marked bradycardia and apnea, as in the dive reflex.

The ventral vagal complex (VVC), unique to mammals, is a recent adaptation to the high oxygen need of this class of animals, and finely tunes energy utilization by subtle and flexible influences on heart rate. The VVC contributes to the initial relatively muted response to arousal, conserving energy until the degree of threat has been determined. Tonic activation of the VVC is inhibited if a significant threat is documented, and is followed by activation of the sympathetic nervous system and mobilization of fight/flight resources. If the mammal is unable to effectively deter the threat through mobilization of sympathetically tuned systems (neuromuscular, cardiovascular), rapid reduction in sympathetic tone may occur. This event is then followed by increase in DVC tone, with marked bradycardia, apnea, sphincter relaxation and gastrointestinal activation. DVC activation mimics the freeze/immobility response, is associated with life-threatening cardiac arrhythmias and bradycardia in mammals, and has perhaps its extreme expression in humans in the phenomenon of voodoo death, as previously described by Cannon.[39] This state, as studied in animals, is associated with death due to cardiac arrest during relaxation or diastole, with the heart flaccid and engorged with blood.[40,41] The extremes of vagal parasympathetic tone therefore contribute greatly to severe emotions, especially those associated with extreme terror and helplessness.

Although the resulting freeze/immobility response may be lifesaving in some cases, recurrent activation of this response as part of the dissociative response in PTSD has clear and serious health and disease implications. As higher levels of adaptation to stress become ineffective, more primitive reflexes no longer useful for survival emerge and exact their toll on the health and survival of the traumatized mammal, and in our case, the human.

Understanding the role of the polyvagal system, as well as endorphins, in dissociation may help to define the relationship of dissociation with the basic primitive freeze response in animals, including the human species. As we have noted, the freeze response is probably mediated by the activation of DVC influences through failure of autonomic sympathetic arousal to effect escape from a life-threatening event. Although cyclical sympathetic/parasympathetic neural and somatic events continue at the onset of the freeze, the victim quickly cycles deep into a state of analgesic immobility mediated by vagal and endorphinergic dominance. This state is characterized by the varying conscious perceptions described at the beginning of this chapter. If traumatization occurs, predicated by the absence of "discharge," or completion of the motor sequences involved in flight, the victim may then manifest variations of reemergence of procedural memory for the experiences of the trauma in the form of dissociative perceptions.

These cognitive and somatic perceptions continue to have ongoing meaning to the survival of the victim, because completion of the act of flight has not occurred. Late somatic dissociation, therefore, represents reexperiencing of survival-based messages, and may be cognitive, perceptual, autonomic, or sensorimotor in expression. I believe that the entire state and experience of dissociation represents an altered state of cognition and somatic perception, driven by attempts to integrate fragments of unresolved traumatic procedural memory, and shaped by the state of increased endorphinergic and vagal tone of the freeze response.

THE CONCEPT OF BOUNDARIES

Not only does the concept of autonomic oscillation in PTSD pertain to the physiology of its specific criteria-based symptoms, but it also relates to the mechanism of somatic and nonphysiological symptoms and findings. With careful observation, one can find clues to perceptual and autonomic changes in regions of the body and the surrounding environment, indicating trauma-based somatic and regional autonomic dysfunction. In this light, let us revisit the concept of boundaries with regard to the perceptual distortions seen in dissociation.

In Chapter 1, we discussed the theoretical concept of perceptual boundaries that guide us in our awareness of our physical sense of self in relation to the outside world. As Joe Kurtz, a psychiatric colleague of mine commented, "The concept of boundaries is to psychology as water is to cooking." The boundaries to which he referred were the intangible areas of sense of self that we perceive in our relationships to others, the regions of subtle limitations in personal and social interaction. Although the concept of boundaries to which I refer includes this concept, mine is a much broader use of the term. Boundaries in my context also include our unconscious proprioceptive awareness of a spatial zone containing a sense of safety and wholeness, not only as it relates to emotions and relationships but also to the tangible, as well as the intangible, material world. It is, in effect, our perceptual surround.

One effect of traumatic stress is to distort or rupture those boundaries, creating a loss of our sense of safety in relation to the world. Boundary rupture occurs not only on a generalized, but also on a regional basis. The resulting sense of perceptual confusion contributes to enhanced arousal, and also to the process of constriction and avoidance seen in PTSD. The other peculiar effect resulting from loss of accurate sense of boundaries is actual physical clumsiness and the tendency to hurt oneself. Many of my MVA-related PTSD patients have experienced repeated minor injuries resulting from what can only be described as clumsiness. When asked about this problem, they invariably excitedly agree that their grace and dexterity have deteriorated. Many such patients experience falls for trivial reasons such as tripping over curbs or objects in their house. They often will bump into objects even in familiar places, especially on the side of the body where somatic dissociation can be documented by "nonphysiological signs." They will slice their fingers preparing food, drop bottles, cups, and pans, break dishes, and drive their spouses to distraction. They seem especially prone to spraining their ankles when stepping off curbs, walking down stairs, or getting out of cars. They seem to be continuously covered with bruises and Band-Aids. I will counsel them with concern about driving, because in addition to injuring themselves during everyday activities, they also are very prone to being involved in further MVAs. This increased risk in traffic probably is related to distraction resulting from dissociation, as well as suppression of attention and visual perception in regions of boundary rupture. These areas of boundary rupture are usually defined and regional, and often are identifiable as developing in the perceptual region where the threat was first identified.

As seen in the patient with a measurable refractive error in one eye due to dissociation, the area of boundary interruption often relates to the region of the perceptual surround where the person first glimpsed or otherwise sensed the threat. The localized area of the body that first experienced an impact or blow, the surrounding area from which the person heard the threatening noise, or the direction in which the body was forcibly thrust might all potentially create an area of impaired boundary continuity. Areas of such changes in perception undoubtedly represent evidence for procedural memory for a threat experienced in that region, leading to a dissociative response in the face of stimuli arising from that area. The generalization of perceived threat from the dissociated region is an example of the tendency for the traumatized individual to become sensitized to increasingly minor and nonspecific sources of arousal.

The presence of localized areas of boundary rupture can also be documented in the clinical treatment setting. As part of our trauma treatment, our therapists prepare patients by seating them in a comfortable reclining chair with their eyes closed. The therapist then quietly walks slowly around the patient and speaks softly from various areas of the perimeter, asking the patient about perceptions and feelings. As the therapist approaches an area of boundary rupture in the patient's perimeter, the patient may experience a sense of arousal or mild anxiety. Physical symptoms associated with this exercise usually are visceral in nature, including a sensation of tightness in the chest, mild nausea, and "a hollow feeling in the pit of the stomach." These physical sensations undoubtedly represent symptoms related to the early mammalian system of arousal involving the ventral vagal complex. These areas of impaired boundary integrity therefore represent regions of potential threat to the patient based on implicit proprioceptive memory for the traumatic event and the region in which it occurred.

I will usually perform a crude test of boundary integrity with my MVA patients. Standing facing the patient, I will slowly move my hand around his or her visual periphery at a distance of about four feet while the patient continues to look at my face. This maneuver will often elicit an arousal response characterized by eye blink, pupillary dilatation, flushing, or even flinching or withdrawal of the body when I reach a specific and reproducible point of visual boundary stimulation. Patients will usually report dizziness, distraction, nausea, or chest constriction at that moment. Occasionally the patient may only experience a vague sense of uneasiness, or in some cases, irritability or a sense of dislike in that region. One can usually relate that area to some meaningful and regional element of the traumatic event, such as being impacted broadside from that direction in an MVA, or assaulted from behind in a mugging or rape. At times this exercise may be so distressing that arousal is only dissipated if the examiner stands at the door, or even across the hallway.

The area of sensitivity to boundary stimulus usually corresponds to an area of the body associated with nonphysiological symptoms or findings, consistent with their dissociative origin. In cases of a history of severe, multiple traumatic experiences, especially sexual abuse as a child, the patient may have *no* areas of visual or perceptual stimulation that are not associated with discomfort or arousal, and the whole exercise of visual or perceptual boundary testing may be intolerable. Caution must be applied with this exercise in such cases.

Finally, boundary ruptures also are identifiable by postural changes that reflect unconscious moving of the body away from the dissociated area by assuming bent or twisted static postures, such as in the patient with arm pain after extensive skin grafts. At times, however, there may be no associated sensorimotor symptoms to identify the area of impaired boundary. For instance, approaching the rape or incest victim from behind in the office examination room, or requesting that the victim lie prone on the table to examine the back may be enough to trigger a panic attack in the absence of regional symptoms. Even without awareness of an alteration in body sensation, arousal may occur with anticipation of kinesthetic, visual, or auditory sensory input to that region of impaired boundary sense. As a result, the victim of trauma with areas of indefensible boundaries will be repetitively subjected to subliminal arousal stimuli that serve to perpetuate autonomic oscillation. The concept of boundary rupture is a useful tool for understanding somatic dissociation, as well as traumatization in general.

SOMATIC DISSOCIATION AND DISEASE

Victims of trauma likely manifest dissociation in these regions of the body as a protection from the arousal triggered by any sensory input from them. A more mysterious and remarkable feature of these areas of somatic dissociation is the presence of subtle signs of autonomic dysfunction affecting the integument, a physical finding that I have documented with increasing frequency as I have explored this phenomenon with my traumatized patients. Many patients with whiplash complain of numbness of the face and head, usually attributed to referred symptoms from the cervical spine, or from myofascial trigger points. Further investigation, however, may reveal a pattern of alternating flushing and pallor, often associated with cyclical swelling of the involved area of the face or scalp. To my great surprise, one patient told me that, according to her hairdresser, her hair grew half an inch less per month on the affected side. This patient had dramatic sensorimotor symptoms affecting the entire right side of her body, associated with nonphysiological physical findings that could only be defined as conversion. Subsequent histories from numerous patients have revealed a frequent, often asymmetrical pattern of hair loss and delayed hair growth in skin areas that were not physically injured in the accident, but which presented with unexplainable sensory symptoms or pain. I have observed abnormally excessive hair growth, erythema, and edema in similar areas of the head, face, or extremities in similar individuals. A few such patients with these types of atypical symptoms in their extremities have experienced progression of signs and symptoms to the point of fulfilling criteria for the diagnosis of sympathetically maintained pain syndromes or reflex sympathetic dystrophy (RSD).

Sympathetically maintained pain, complex regional pain, and RSD are relatively common, unexplained painful syndromes characterized by severe pain associated with regional vasomotor symptoms and signs, both parasympathetic and sympathetic in nature. They constitute a spectrum of pain syndromes associated with vasomotor signs of which RSD is the extreme expression. RSD is associated with unusual burning, intolerable pain that often follows traumatic physical injuries, but may also follow trivial physical trauma (see Chapter 9 for references and further discussion). The use of the term "sympathetic" in reference to this diagnosis relates to the predominance of vasoconstrictive and dystrophic symptoms and signs that characterize the later stages of the syndrome. In fact, trophic or parasympathetic signs, including hair growth and erythema, may accompany the early phases of the syndrome. In its worst forms, the affected region of the body may develop hair loss, dystonic flexor contractures, and atrophy of skin, muscles, bone, and connective tissue. In rare cases, the symptoms of intolerable burning pain may spread to contiguous or remote areas of the body. Milder forms of the condition have prompted the division of diagnostic subcategories to include the designations of complex regional pain syndrome, and sympathetically maintained pain. In some cases, actual cyclical vascular autonomic changes are apparent.

The cause of this perplexing condition has defied explanation, and both central and peripheral neurogenic causes have been proposed. An intriguing recent study of the H-reflex in dystonia related to end-stage RSD suggests the influence of supraspinal, or central brain mechanisms, in the etiology of this posture.[42] The authors actually state, "In causalgia-dystonia, central motor control may be altered by a trauma in such a way that the affected limb is dissociated from normal regulatory mechanisms"[42] (p. 2198). I would propose the theory that RSD is a continuum, ranging from the most subtle of autonomic symptoms in a dissociated body region to the full-blown intractable pain syndrome that has been classically described.

Both RSD and the regional autonomic syndrome that I have described have sympathetic and parasympathetic signs, with the sympathetic findings ultimately predominating. RSD occurs most commonly after a particularly traumatic physical injury, and patients who develop RSD may have a higher incidence of prior life trauma. The pattern of pain and sensory loss in RSD is occasionally dermatomal, but more often is in a linear "nonphysiological stocking and glove" distribution in the extremities, much like that seen in conversion or dissociation. The autonomic nervous system is distributed in a linear fashion in many parts of the body, along the pathways of the peripheral vascular system, rather than in the layered, dermatomal pattern of the somatic peripheral nervous system. This more linear pattern of distribution of autonomic nerves may at least partially explain the linear "nonphysiological" pattern of sensory loss in both conversion and RSD.

I believe that the phenomenon of regional somatic dissociation is directly linked to the freeze, or dissociative response, occurring at the moment of a traumatic event in a state of helplessness. Just as in myofascial pain, the implicit and procedural memory for both motor and proprioceptive messages accessed at the moment of trauma is stored, in this case powerfully so, under the influence of input from amygdala, brainstem motor nuclei, and regional cortical centers. Unless the experience related to the traumatic event is dissipated through completion of the physiological cycle of trauma by intense motor activity, the sensorimotor features of that traumatic stress will be imprinted in implicit memory through basic operant conditioning, to be accessed in the future for the purpose of survival.

Pain perception will be especially powerfully imprinted. In unresolved traumatic stress dissociation will cause fragmentation and distortion of the traumatic memories accompanying the event, including any pain associated with it. Therefore, the "objective" manifestations of that injury will likewise be distorted and non-physiological. Abnormally severe allodynia in trauma not only reflects the injury, but also the threat associated with it, with the pain becoming part of the sensory input from the original threat. Thus, one often notes apparent pain exaggeration related to limited objective pathology in traumatized patients and specifically in those with unexplained chronic pain. The linkage of that pain to implicit memory in trauma associated with dissociation may well explain many of the instances of chronic pain that are no longer explainable by imaging techniques or physical findings. As in many unexplainable symptoms, the *meaning* of the pain with regard to survival in the face of life-threatening traumatic stress may hold the key to understanding its persistence after the apparent physical cause has been "cured" by current medical standards. The root of chronic pain in this model lies in conditioned implicit pain memory as a reflection of traumatic imprinting.

Pain "memory" may be viewed as a defensive survival tool in the face of an unresolved threat, a conditioned survival response and perception rendered ineffectual because the physiological response of freeze/dissociation has literally blocked the survival brain from instinctively "realizing" that the threat is over. In RSD, however, that pain is associated with variable, but consistent regional autonomic symptoms and signs. I believe that RSD represents the extreme of traumatic pain memory based on the severity of the dissociative response accompanying the traumatic stress. The region of the body experiencing the pain and now representing a perceived threat has been dissociated in much the same way that a threatening memory may be dissociated in traumatic amnesia. Exposure of this dissociated region of the body to the abnormal oscillation of autonomic tone in trauma results in regional autonomic dysregulation, fluctuating signs of abnormal parasympathetic and sympathetic tone, and the variable syndromes of complex regional pain and RSD. Ultimately, the mechanism of tissue injury and disease in this model is sustained vasoconstriction to the point of ischemic damage to the tissue of the dissociated body region.

This pathophysiological phenomenon of dissociation, autonomic dysregulation, and vasoconstriction provides a compelling etiologic rationale for many of the diseases of unknown cause that are linked epidemiologically to traumatic stress. Syndromes of smooth muscle spasm and/or ulceration in the gastrointestinal system are associated with chronic stress exposure in most cases. These include esophageal cardiospasm, gastroesophageal reflux disease, peptic ulcer disease, ulcerative colitis, regional ileitis, and irritable bowel syndrome. Interstitial cystitis is associated with painful bladder ulcers and symptoms of motor dyssynergia of the bladder, also of unknown cause. Classic migraine, of course, is a prototypical example of vascular manifestations of autonomic cyclical dysregulation, and has been linked to prior trauma in a number of recent studies.[43-45] Many of these conditions have been linked to characterological features of personality development suggesting a common behavioral and developmental basis, in keeping with Schore's theories of neonatal brain development and susceptibility to later psychopathology and physical disease.[37]

In addition, many chronic diseases by their very nature are a *source* of trauma, since by definition they constitute a threat to life in a state of helplessness, that state of vulnerability produced in no small part by the frustrating failure of current medical science to effectively treat chronic disease. As we shall see in Chapter 9, cancer and heart disease are associated with a significant and largely unappreciated incidence of PTSD. I believe therefore that cumulative life trauma and its associated autonomic dysfunction may not only contribute to the development of selective chronic diseases, but may also contribute to the progression of these diseases through similar processes, probably analogous to the kindling model of PTSD.

CONCLUSION

The phenomenon of dissociation may be the most critical element of traumatization. Dissociation, or freeze, at the moment of trauma is perhaps the main defining event in the development of subsequent PTSD. It may well account for many of the cognitive deficits attributed to a physical closed head injury in selected cases. The neurochemical and neurophysiological correlates of dissociation include endorphinergic neural effects, changes in HPA dynamics, and marked autonomic lability in the form of abnormal oscillatory cycling between extremes of sympathetic and parasympathetic tone. These forces may well be the engine driving the kindled brain circuitry of PTSD.

The concept of somatic dissociation as a tangible and clinically measurable change in regional autonomic physiology challenges current concepts of the criteria for somatization and somatiform disorders, conversion disorder, and pain disorder. As defined in the DSM-IV, all of these disorders cannot be fully explained by a known medical condition, or the direct effect of a substance.[31] On the contrary, we believe that these conditions, as subsets of dissociation, are actually defined by demonstrable vasomotor changes in the dissociated regions of the body. It is not enough to say that somatization reflects expression of an emotion in a somatic symptom, or that conversion represents a symptom in the absence of a medical condition. Rather, psychosomatic syndromes appear to reflect subtle but demonstrable physiological changes in dissociated regional end organs based on changes in autonomic tone, dependent in turn on trauma-related central and autonomic nervous system kindled responses, and mediated by vasoconstriction.

These concepts may have a correlate in other unexplained medical phenomena. In phantom limb pain, implicit memory for trauma-related pain persists in the form of altered perception even though the injured part has literally been dismembered. In shoulder-hand syndrome, related to the marked alteration in sensory perception of an arm in a stroke, the hand and arm may develop progressive and painful dystrophic contractures in an apparently anesthetic limb.[46,47] In somatic dissociation, the area of the body representing the trauma-related threat is perceptually dissociated, disembodied, and also literally dismembered. Isolation of a body part from normal perception, whether by brain injury, traumatic procedural memory, or dissociation, appears to affect the basic nutrition of that region, perhaps by altered autonomic regulation as discussed in the body of this chapter. I believe these phenomena are of critical importance to the understanding of many chronic diseases of unknown cause, and may have a major bearing on the progression of any chronic disease.

Unless one closely examines the traumatized patient for these objective physical findings, the somatic manifestations of dissociation may confuse and frustrate the medical professional attempting to treat the patient's physical complaints. Close inspection of regions of somatic dissociation may allow the clinician to gain insight into the sometimes subtle, but meaningful, objective autonomic changes in the involved areas of the body. Only by understanding the mechanism and somatic manifestations of dissociation in each individual can one begin to develop an effective mode of treatment. Unless one is able to break through, extinguish, or quench the dissociative component of PTSD, effective treatment may be frustrated for the emotional components of PTSD and the unexplained chronic pain, somatic syndromes, and chronic diseases that often accompany traumatic stress.

Chapter 9

Sources of Trauma

Joan was referred to me by her physical therapist, who thought that Joan might be suffering from PTSD. As she walked into my office, I noted that she held her left hand in a strange dystonic and flexed position, that her eyes squinted in the fluorescent lighting, and that she spoke slowly with a stutter. Her thoughts were scattered, and it took her almost ten minutes to state that her symptoms had begun two months before, following postmastectomy breast reconstruction surgery. During that procedure, she had awakened shortly after anesthetic induction to find herself helpless, paralyzed, blindfolded, intubated, and fully conscious while the surgeon made his first incision. Thereafter, she remained fully awake while she listened to conversations of the operating room staff, and felt every painful detail of the opening and manipulation of her body by knives and forceps. She made every effort of will to alert the staff to her conscious state, but EEGs, cardiac monitors, and her blood gas levels gave no clue to her being awake. Toward the end of the ninety-minute operation, she began to hallucinate, and really felt little pain, although she still recalls the content of conversation in the room during the procedure and the coldness of the water used to irrigate her wound. As drugs and tubes were removed at the end, and the paralysis cleared, her muscles involuntarily went into such violent contractions against the restraints used in the surgery that she had massive bruises for weeks thereafter on her arms and legs.

In the ensuing weeks, she predictably developed acute PTSD, with flashbacks, nightmares of knives and wounds, panic, intrusive thoughts, confusion, and severe cognitive problems. Remarkably, she also developed all of the physical symptoms of whiplash, with vertigo, loss of balance, sound and light sensitivity, severe nocturnal bruxism, cervical myofascial pain, headaches, and ocular convergence insufficiency. Her surgeon suggested that the experience might have been a dream, and believed that her symptoms would go away with time. Her posture was quite dramatic, and was manifested by a position of flexion, dystonia, and defensive infolding of the left arm, head, and shoulder, as if protecting her left chest area from assault.

* * *

Studies addressing the epidemiology of trauma and post-traumatic stress disorder have been substantially influenced by the definitions of these terms in the *Diagnostic and Statistical Manual of Mental Disorders* (DSM)-III, -III(R), and -IV. Standardization of terms is necessary if one is to arrive at any statistical consistency when attempting to determine the frequency of an event or condition. Revision of the definitions of trauma and PTSD through the sequential editions of the DSM over the past fifteen years undoubtedly has affected the ability of researchers to compare the incidence of these conditions.[1,2,3] An early study of PTSD in 1987 estimated an incidence in the general population of 1 percent.[4] As the clinical syndrome seen in response to a traumatic event became clearer, and the definition of that event became more inclusive of a wider range of societal experiences, the incidence of PTSD has predictably increased. Based on current definitions of trauma and PTSD, estimates of PTSD in the general population range from 3 to 6 percent.[5] It is becoming increasingly clear, however, that the true incidence of traumatization and the late syndromes of PTSD are vastly underestimated by these statistics.

Early recognition of traumatization in individuals was associated almost exclusively with war-related experiences. Such terms as "shell shock" and "battle fatigue" reflected this association. Eventually it became apparent that a relatively broad spectrum of experiences could lead to a group of symptoms comparable to those experienced in combat. Early responses to this association led to such diagnoses as "situational maladjustment," "gross stress reactions," and "adjustment disorders" in the *International Statistical Classification of Diseases, Injuries and Causes of Death* (ICD, revisions 6, 8, and 9), and the DSM-I-II.[6,7] It was not until 1980 that the term PTSD was introduced in the DSM-III.

The concept of the intrinsic difference between stress and a traumatic event has also evolved along with the interpretation of the individual's response to such events. Stress has long been known to exert a marked and, at times, injurious effect on the body and to produce a pattern of predictable emotional responses. However, a stressful event alone is unlikely to produce the relatively stereotyped and long-lasting symptoms of PTSD in a healthy individual. The DSM-IV clearly implies that only a relatively catastrophic event will predictably elicit the syndrome of PTSD. Such an event would require that the individual "experienced, witnessed, or was confronted with an event or events that involved actual death or serious injury, or a threat to the physical integrity of self or others"[3] (p. 427). In addition, the person's response to that event should involve "intense fear, helplessness, or horror"[3] (p. 428). As I proposed in Chapter 1, however, the meaning of the event to the person exposed to it might well create an environment sufficiently threatening to constitute an adequate criterion for the above definition, even though another person might not experience a similar event as traumatic. The female victim of incest or rape predictably might develop acute PTSD after an experience of transient fondling on a crowded bus, whereas a previously nontraumatized female might respond with anger and fear, but not dissociation. As previously noted, in my experiences with relatively trivial low velocity MVAs, victims of substantial prior trauma may respond with a full-blown whiplash syndrome, including PTSD, despite the definition of this type of trauma not approaching the DSM-IV criteria. The somatic expressions of the whiplash syndrome, in fact, may represent a universal constellation of symptoms attributable to recurrent activation by procedural memory of the instinctive defensive response to *any* unresolved life-threatening experience. This dichotomy is extremely important in the assessment of what constitutes forms and sources of trauma in our society. The special meaning of the threat to the victim based on his or her past experience must be considered before dismissing the threat as not sufficient to be traumatizing.

In addition, criteria for the diagnosis of PTSD require one or more patterns of reexperiencing, three or more of avoidance, and two or more of arousal. This type of threshold requirement for establishing the diagnosis of PTSD is probably necessary for standardization, but creates an artificial barrier to the diagnosis of traumatization. The expression of symptoms of trauma is not rigidly set, but composes a continuum based on the type and severity of the trauma, the past experience of the victim, the prevalence of dissociation, age, gender, and many other factors. Incomplete criteria based on the DSM-IV must not imply that the victims have not been traumatized by the experience, and that the basis for their expressed symptoms is not PTSD. In the area of PTSD associated with MVAs, Blanchard and Hickling have proposed a "subsyndromal" form of PTSD in an attempt to address this dilemma.[8] The obvious risk of arbitrarily broadening the clinical definition of symptoms of trauma is loss of the standardization required for developing a legitimate statistical epidemiological base. On the other hand, ignoring the somatic symptoms of trauma based on dissociation, and of the many subsyndromal expressions of trauma, creates an inappropriately limited appreciation of the disastrous effects of life trauma on our societal health.

Van der Kolk and colleagues have explored the significance of dissociation, affect dysregulation, and somatization as "associated features" of PTSD.[9] They studied three groups of patients: those currently fulfilling diagnostic criteria for PTSD, those with lifelong PTSD but not currently meeting criteria, and those with no PTSD. Among other findings, they specifically noted that the "associated features" often persisted for years, even after full-blown PTSD symptoms have subsided. An important implication of their study is that subsidence of acute PTSD symptoms sufficient to make the criteria-based diagnosis of PTSD no longer tenable ignores the long-term, pervasive, and often somatic consequences of exposure to traumatic stress. These "associated disorders," and indeed many of the diseases of trauma (Chapter 9), must be considered to be part of the continuum of the diffuse physiological changes initiated by a traumatic event, and associated initially with the syndrome of PTSD. For this reason, although I will review statistical data regarding the relative incidence of various sources of life trauma, I will also explore the theoretical basis for other predictable but relatively unexplored traumatic societal events and experiences.

THE DEFINITION OF TRAUMATIC STRESS

Any consideration of the relative incidence of PTSD after specific types of traumatic events obviously depends directly on the accepted criteria for an event having the potential to be traumatizing. Levine would define trauma as any event that produced the requisite physiological event—in his model, an unresolved freeze response, or dissociation.[10] Several other investigators have taken a similar theoretical direction based on the response of the individual to trauma. Krystal has suggested that psychic surrender, or "freezing of the affect" may represent a typical response to extreme stress.[11] Hobfoll also suggests that the response of resource conservation, or "playing dead," may imply exposure to a severe stress sufficient to qualify as traumatic stress.[12]

The American Psychiatric Association, in the DSM-III-R, defined a traumatic event as one "that is outside the range of usual human experience and that would be markedly distressing to almost anyone"[2] (p. 250). This definition does not imply that a specific behavioral or physiological response to the experience is essential, as suggested previously. In the DSM-IV, a traumatic event is defined as "The person experienced, witnessed, or was confronted with an event or events that involved actual or threatened death or serious injury"[3] (p. 427). In addition, the experience of helplessness or horror is added to the definition, thereby incorporating the response of the individual to the event. Breslau and Davis, and Solomon and Canino would agree with the need to define traumatic stress more by the response elicited by it than by a conceptual definition of the event itself.[13,14] By their definition, any stressor sufficient to produce the traumatic symptoms of reexperiencing, arousal, and avoidance should qualify as a traumatic event. Norris, on the other hand, has introduced the concept of violence, involving sudden extreme force from an external agent, as a reasonable source of traumatic stress.[15] Designed primarily for research, Norris's concept would include events related to nature, technology, and human behavior as sources of trauma. Like Blanchard and Hickling,[8] she also notes that the limiting constraints of the DSM-IV criteria results in a definition of PTSD that ". . . represents only the tip of the iceberg in terms of experienced distress"[15] (p. 416). She further states, "In reporting rates of disorder that are constrained to be low, one should be cautious not to give the mistaken impression that few people become distressed following traumatic events"[15] (p. 416).

One would have difficulty with the conclusion that traumatic stress had occurred without a sufficient behavioral and physiological response to an event. The spectrum of such responses clearly varies widely between individuals: people are primed to respond to a variety of stressful events based on a myriad of predisposing factors. What may produce surprise and perhaps consternation in one individual may induce shock and dissociation in another. The potential for an event to be traumatizing depends in part on the meaning of the event to the person experiencing it. This assumption, however, has not been entirely supported by researchers in PTSD. The DSM-III concluded that PTSD is a normal response caused by an abnormal incident, and would be expected to occur in the majority of people experiencing that incident.[1] Much of the PTSD literature does not allow for the concept that a full-blown and prolonged traumatic physiological response may occur after a relatively minor stressful event if the victim has a past history of severe trauma, especially as a child.

My experience in hundreds of cases has been that childhood trauma may produce a state of sensitization, vulnerability, or diminished reserve capacity to stress that may result in an overwhelming physiological stress response and full-blown clinical PTSD in response to a nonspecific societal stress such as a trivial MVA. I strongly support those authors who feel that the response of the victim to a traumatically stressful event is the defining factor for traumatization, taking into careful account that individual's life burden of traumatic stress. I also maintain that the definition of a recognized response to traumatic stress must include not only those symptoms related to reexperiencing, arousal, and avoidance defined in the DSM-IV, but also must address comorbid, associated, and somatic symptoms known to be related to past exposure to trauma.

EXPOSURE TO COMBAT

As we have noted, most of the early studies in trauma arose from experiences with victims of traumatic stress related to wartime combat experiences. From shell shock in World War I to battle fatigue in World War II, researchers in trauma derived many of their observations and theories from the study of wartime veterans experiencing emotional distress based on their exposure to combat. The term "combat stress reaction" (CSR) eventually was applied to the acute behavioral, emotional, and physical symptoms seen in some soldiers exposed to combat.[16] These symptoms constitute a complex and variable mix that reflect the linking of psychological and somatic complaints seen in late PTSD, some of which are ignored in the DSM-IV. Agitation, increased startle, stimulus sensitivity, and irritability reflect increased arousal. Apathy, depression, and psychomotor retardation may alternate with increased arousal; somatic, and primarily autonomic, symptoms may include nausea, diarrhea and constipation, and abdominal cramping.[17]

Exposure to combat-related traumatic stress in the Vietnam War was not likely to have been more severe than in the previous great wars. The controversial nature of the Vietnam conflict and the difficulties with societal assimilation of many returning veterans, however, may have sensitized the scientific community to the distress evidenced in many members of the military who experienced combat there. Increased awareness of the emotional burden carried by these soldiers has led to extensive follow-up studies, which have yielded a great deal of data regarding PTSD, have led to the term PTSD itself, and have helped to define the syndrome as we now know it. Much of the early data came from the National Vietnam Veterans Readjustment Study (NVVRS), from which the study *Trauma and the Vietnam War Generation* was published.[18] At the time of the latter study, using DSM-III-R criteria, 15.2 percent of then current male Vietnam War veterans suffered from PTSD, and 11 percent from partial PTSD. The number of veterans who had a lifetime prevalence that included prior experience of criteria-based symptoms was 30.9 percent. Lifetime prevalence implies the presence of symptoms sufficient to diagnose PTSD at any time in their lives. A National Comorbidity Survey (NCS) by Kessler and colleagues estimated that the risk of developing PTSD after exposure to combat is 38.8 percent.[19] Epidemiological studies of the occurrence of PTSD in the Vietnam War clearly reflect a substantial incidence of combat-related PTSD in wartime, based on relatively strict DSM-III-R criteria. These findings of a relatively high incidence of the development of criteria-based PTSD after exposure to the experience of war-related combat are certainly predictable based on the emergence of this diagnosis from the theater of war.

These findings, however, do not necessarily reflect the breadth of varied and long-term symptoms that may occur long after criteriabase PTSD or CSR has subsided. Late problems in combat veterans experiencing CSR include impaired performance in work-related, family-related, sexual, and social functioning that does not appear to improve with time.[16] Increased somatic complaints, poorer indices of health and attempts at health maintenance have been reported in veterans who have experienced CSR.[20-22] Some Persian Gulf War veterans (PGV) returned from combat with a somatic syndrome consisting of myalgias, arthralgias, headache, weakness, pathological fatigue, memory loss, sleep disorders, skin rashes, hair loss, dyspnea, and gastrointestinal complaints.[23-25] In the majority of these cases, physical diagnostic explanations have included asthma, migraines, and inflammatory bowel symptoms of unknown cause.[25] Psychiatric explanations have included PTSD, anxiety disorder, and depression.[25] Approximately 15 percent have remained unexplained.[23-25] Amato and colleagues studied neuromuscular symptoms in PGVs and found no objective evidence of neuromuscular disease.[26] They commented on the remarkable similarity of symptoms in these PGVs to fibromyalgia and chronic fatigue syndrome, noting that many of their patients also suffered from anxiety, headaches, depression, sleep disturbance, and bowel disorders. We are once again presented with the dilemma of an unexplained somatic/psychological symptom complex clearly following exposure to traumatic stress. When one is locked into the confining definitions of the DSM-IV and adherence to Cartesian dualism, such syndromes defy explanation. When viewed outside of these constraints, however, they fall into the logical niche of trauma-based psychophysiological pathology (see Chapter 6).

Within the group of soldiers who develop PTSD, a number of factors seemed to contribute to their vulnerability. Bremner and colleagues found that a history of childhood physical abuse appeared to be a significant contributory factor to the development of PTSD in Vietnam veterans.[27] They concluded that exposure to prior trauma was not protective in dealing with a new traumatic event, but might even increase vulnerability to further traumatization. This conclusion is quite in keeping with my observations concerning increased vulnerability to traumatic stress in motor vehicle accidents when a person has a prior history of trauma, especially when it has occurred in childhood. A number of studies have documented that Vietnam veterans suffering from PTSD differed from their non-PTSD cohorts in their lack of support from postwar social systems, including that from spouses, family members, and fellow veterans.[28-31] These studies, however, were unable to differentiate whether development and perpetuation of PTSD were enhanced by the lack of social support, or whether avoidance as a symptomatic component of PTSD led to social isolation, and therefore lack of support. Intensity of combat exposure is a predictable factor in the development of PTSD, and this conclusion is supported by many studies.[28-32] Although these studies provide only a few clues to the sources of vulnerability to CSR and PTSD, they support the presence of diminished reserve capacity and resiliency in trauma associated with a history of prior traumatic stress. They also emphasize the importance of the availability of adequate support systems after trauma.

CHILD ABUSE

The well-documented association of childhood psychological, physical, and sexual abuse with a remarkable constellation of somatic symptoms in adulthood, also strongly supports the link between a traumatic emotional experience and subsequent somatic dysfunction. Child abuse has been linked to a wide variety of chronic and often unexplained pain syndromes, including pelvic, low back, orofacial, and bladder pain, as well as fibromyalgia. Irritable bowel syndrome, interstitial cystitis, anorexia, and bulimia have all been linked to child abuse, especially sexual abuse (see Chapter 6).

The vulnerability of the developing brain to positive and negative affective experiences has been thoroughly explored in recent years, and provides a solid neurophysiological substrate for the development of adaptive and maladaptive changes in brain morphology and function.[33,34] These changes in turn will likely affect not only autonomic adaptations to further stressors, but also promote the development of somatic physiological changes that will predispose the adult survivor of childhood trauma to predictable physical disease and behavioral dysfunction. Exposure to traumatic stress in childhood is particularly likely to result in long-lasting and varied late symptoms of trauma. Traumatic stress at any age produces persistent, and at times, permanent changes in brain structure and chemistry. Exposure to trauma will predictably have a far more profound effect on the developing brain of the infant or very young child, producing permanent patterns of neuronal development that may result in specific disturbances in personality and behavior.[34,35]

Infants and young children, especially females, are especially susceptible to dissociate, or freeze in the face of trauma (see Chapter 8). Males are much more likely to become activated, and enter the fight/flight continuum. This is clearly reflected in the predominance of aggressive, hyperactive, and acting-out behavior in disturbed boys, and the converse tendency for traumatized girls to manifest depression, anxiety, or borderline personality traits. The benefit of aggression in males and freeze/dissociation in females in the face of threat for species survival is obvious.[34] Dissociation in male members of the tribe in the face of danger would preclude the defensive behavior on which the tribe is dependent. Aggressive behavior on the part of physically weaker children or females would jeopardize their survival. This dichotomy is illustrated by the remarkable incidence of a past history of child abuse in prison populations, especially among males, where violent behavior has led to incarceration.[36] In fourteen male juvenile murderers condemned to death in 1987, Lewis and colleagues noted that twelve had been severely physically abused and five had suffered sodomy at the hands of their relatives.[37]

Children traumatized when very young, however, are more likely to manifest symptoms of avoidance, constriction, withdrawal, and further dissociation in the future, especially in the face of episodes of traumatic stress (see Chapter 8). Symptoms in the categories of arousal and reexperiencing, and behaviors reflecting these states, are less likely to present themselves in these children, and therefore the criteria-based diagnosis of PTSD may be more difficult to make in this subpopulation.

In one study of severely traumatized children with symptoms of hyperarousal, only 70 percent met DSM-IV criteria for PTSD.[38] Part of the explanation for this discrepancy may be that many of the late symptoms of trauma in children are secondary to dissociation, and present as comorbid disorders that may not reflect their origin in traumatic stress. Symptoms of *hypo*arousal, in fact, may predominate in traumatized children.[9] The diagnostic category Disorders of Stress, Not Otherwise Specified (DESNOS), reflects symptoms associated with self-regulation, impulse control, self-esteem, relationships with others, and dissociative tendencies. Although DESNOS is not recognized as a diagnostic entity by the American Psychiatric Association, one study found that DESNOS as a diagnostic criteria in adult survivors of child abuse correlated more accurately with a poor treatment outcome than did the diagnosis of PTSD based on the DSM-IV.[39] The constraints presented by this dilemma make any attempts at documenting the incidence of traumatic stress and PTSD in children who have experienced abuse extremely difficult if conclusions and diagnostic categorizations are based on DSM-IV criteria.

Problems in estimating the actual incidence of societal child abuse arise from the intrinsic effect of dissociation on traumatic memory. By definition, dissociation may result in fugue-related amnesia for the traumatic event, and although the validity of recovered memories for remote or childhood trauma has been challenged, there is no question that traumatic amnesia is common in childhood.[40] In addition, most adults traumatized as children will not voluntarily divulge this information to their physician.[41] The phenomenon of "effort after meaning," on the other hand, may contribute to amplification of the statistical frequency of child abuse.[42] "Effort after meaning" refers to the tendency for patients who exhibit somatization to search for a reason for their symptoms, especially when confronted with a skeptical medical profession.

Controlling for ethnic, geographic, economic, and cultural variables in studied populations is extremely difficult. Based on these and other factors, it is not surprising that estimates of the societal incidence of child abuse vary widely. In a review of the literature, Wood notes an incidence of childhood sexual abuse in females of between 12 and 64 percent, and in males of 3 and 13 percent.[43] A study from the National Victim Center reported 2,936,00 children in the United States to have been abused or neglected that year.[44] These statistics undoubtedly reflect the varied populations studied, as well as other factors noted previously. Taking all of these factors into consideration, however, the prevalence of child abuse in our society is remarkable and shocking. Many of the late diseases of trauma reflect the sustained autonomic dysregulation linked specifically to dissociation. Adult survivors of child abuse bear a legacy of altered physiological responsiveness and resulting susceptibility to a wide spectrum of chronic diseases (see Chapters 6 and 8). The emotional, physical, social, and economic toll on our society from the shattered lives of our abused children is far more widespread and overwhelming than we currently seem to realize.

Victims of prior child abuse present one of the most challenging populations to treat for the injuries suffered in a motor vehicle accident. Since dissociation characterizes the basic response to trauma in these individuals, they usually will relate significant symptoms of dissociation at the time of the accident. These symptoms will often persist for weeks, and the associated confusion and numbing will frequently be interpreted as a brain injury. As dissociation subsides, cyclical arousal in the form of emotional lability and anxiety will appear, along with symptoms of full-blown PTSD. These patients usually develop dissociative somatic symptoms that present in a nonphysiological and bizarre fashion. Such symptoms often are linked to arousal and panic, enhancing their perceived severity. Attempts to link dissociative somatic symptoms to spinal injury or other physical causes are usually fruitless. Efforts to treat these symptoms with physical therapeutic measures often are ineffective, or may aggravate them. Intrinsic autonomic instability and other neurochemical and neurophysiological changes intrinsic to dissociation and PTSD often are associated with pharmacological intolerance. Headache and myofascial pain are often intractable, and may respond only to narcotics, which present a problem because narcotics, with their enhancement of endor- phinergic tone, may potentiate dissociation (see Chapter 8). Somatic and highly interactive forms of psychotherapy must be used with great care because of the risk of flooding and resultant dissociation in these individuals. Clearly, the most dramatic examples of severe morbidity and delayed recovery in whiplash fall into the category of those patients with a prior history of child abuse.

SOCIETAL TRAUMA

The risks of exposure to catastrophic and traumatic events occurring in any urban society are predictably high. Victimization by crime in any form can be traumatizing. Even being subjected to personal or financial loss through nonviolent means may prove threatening to one's future through loss of financial security, and the resulting threat to one's physical well-being. The death of a loved one, close friend, or an otherwise important figure in one's life may be threatening enough to induce helplessness. Such personal losses through nonviolent means are generally accepted in our society as inevitable and therefore not felt to be relevant to the concept of traumatic stress. As part of our basically Calvinistic upbringing in the United States, we are encouraged to "suck it up," get over it, and move on in life in the face of pain and loss. Yet, numerous studies support the concern that prior life traumatic events and psychiatric morbidity are associated with a higher risk of developing PTSD after a new trauma, and that this vulnerability may result in an enhanced traumatic reaction even with less intense traumatic exposure.[45-47] As a result, even minor, nonviolent societal trauma should not be dismissed as a source of significant trauma in selected populations.

In general, however, the degree of exposure and intensity of the trauma tend to correlate directly with the incidence and severity of resulting depression and PTSD.[48,49] The literature clearly reveals that there is no shortage of social and natural exposure to extreme stress and trauma throughout the world. The National Comorbidity Study reveals an incidence of exposure to traumatic events in 60.7 percent of the men, and 51.2 percent of the women.[50] Resnick and colleagues, in a national study of adult women in the United States, found a high incidence of exposure to trauma: 35.6 percent had experienced some type of crime, 14.3 percent molestation or sexual assault, 13.4 percent a death of a relative or close friend by murder, 12.7 percent a completed rape, and 10.3 percent a physical assault.[51] Norris found a 69 percent incidence of exposure to a traumatic event in a sample of 1,000 adults in the United States.[52]

Natural and manmade disasters are a worldwide norm. Between 1967 and 1991, disasters killed 7 million people and affected 3 billion.[53] In 1999, the world's attention was riveted on the genocide in Bosnia and in Kosovo. American parents of school-aged children were shocked by the recent emergence of seemingly unprovoked massacres of children in schools throughout the nation by their disturbed peers. In Littleton, Colorado, twelve high school children and one teacher were shot to death by two students who had been ridiculed for their style of dress and lifestyles. The world as a whole is a dangerous place, and neither economic development nor accultura-tion has changed that fact.

Of all of the forms of social trauma, sexual assault, particularly rape, has the greatest potential for leading to PTSD.[54,55] Breslau has documented that most forms of social trauma have a roughly similar potential to elicit symptoms of PTSD, with risk ranging from about 10 to 30 percent.[54] These include physical assault, serious accident or injury, sudden death of a close friend or relative, seeing someone se-riously injured or killed, or a threat to one's life. In Breslau's study, rape and sexual assault are associated with a subsequent incidence of PTSD of 60 percent or more. Koss and Burkhart note that the appear-ance of PTSD symptoms after rape may be delayed for years.[55] They also emphasize the unique implications of sexual assault with regard to the woman's sense of hopelessness and despair. As noted in Chap-ter 1, the magnitude of a traumatic event, and its threat to life, is di-rectly proportional to the meaning of that threat within its societal frame of reference. Threats from primary caregivers are of the great-est magnitude, and physical and sexual assault of children by parents have the potential for the greatest traumatization and subsequent symptoms of trauma. Trauma inflicted by another human being is high on the continuum of severity, and sexual trauma is at the top of that list.

The trauma of rape is predominantly experienced by women, with about 10 percent of rape victims being men, although that figure may be low based on the reluctance of men to report or seek counseling for rape.[56] The act of sexual intercourse in mammalian species is charac-terized by submission of the female to a variable degree, and the ac-ceptance of a state of relative vulnerability, driven by deep-seated instinctual roles governing the survival of the species. In the human species, intercourse has taken on a deep interpersonal meaning in the form of trust, sharing, and accepted vulnerability on the part of the woman. Violation of that state in the form of sexual assault destroys any sense of safe boundaries for that woman within human society, especially in relationship to males. The sense of degradation, guilt, and worthlessness that often accompanies rape is amplified by our society's tendency to doubt the credibility of the victim, to assume complicity in the act, or to imply provocation by the victim. An arti-cle in the international press in 1999 reported that a judge in an Italian court dismissed a rape conviction because the victim wore jeans, a presumed sexually provocative act. Rape myths of this sort in our society continue to perpetuate the fears of reporting the assault by the rape victim. The system of justice that accompanies sexual assault contributes greatly to the victims' sense of helplessness accompanying the event, and potentiates the likelihood of their developing PTSD.

Many cases of rape involve a man with whom the victim is familiar, either in the context of a consensual social event (date rape), or by a familiar acquaintance, friend, or family member. Familiarity with the perpetrator also enhances the sense of betrayal of trust and may increase the intensity of the trauma. Rape by an acquaintance is far more common than by a stranger. In a study of 6,100 undergraduate men and women, Warshaw noted that one out of four women had experienced rape or an attempted rape, 84 percent were acquainted with the rapist, and 57 percent of the rapes occurred on dates.[56] Comparison of the perception of the experience of rape by women who were victims of stranger versus acquaintance rape reveals remarkable differences. Victims of acquaintance rape were more likely not to consider the experience to be rape, and less likely to discuss it with someone, report it to the police, or seek crisis counseling.[57]

The event currently termed "date rape" illustrates this dilemma. In this circumstance, the woman has not only tacitly accepted at least a temporary relationship of trust, but has apparently entered willingly into a date, a presumably mutually pleasurable event. Current societal mores have probably contributed to problems with differentiating what constitutes rape and what constitutes consensual sex in this environment. The sexual revolution of the 1960s supposedly freed women from American society's unilateral expectations of feminine chastity. In reality, these new sexual mores also introduced a new set of expectations regarding the woman's role in friendships and dating relationships with men. The victim of date or acquaintance rape faces a greatly enhanced sense of shame, betrayal, and helplessness considering the fact that she has voluntarily entered a state of vulnerability, and that sexual intimacy may well be an acceptable outcome of the date experience. The sense of guilt resulting from this dilemma enhances her sense of helplessness, and prevents her access to therapy that might mitigate posttraumatic symptoms. In the confusion over the role she may have taken in the assault, the victim of acquaintance rape often will tend to assume some responsibility for the event. She may blame herself, have doubts about whether the event was indeed rape, and hesitate to file a police report or tell anyone about it. As one patient of mine put it, "I had sex lots of times in college when I didn't want to because I was too ashamed to refuse it. Now that I think back, a couple of times it was rape." Without the victim experiencing and expressing the normal rage associated with the assault under these circumstances, the dissociation so often reported by rape victims will continue to recur and to perpetuate the late emotional and somatic symptoms of trauma. Hesitancy by acquaintance rape victims to report assaults probably contributes to a much higher rate of rape and sexual assault than is reflected by current statistics.

In my experience with whiplash patients who have a past history of rape, delayed recovery with emotional and somatic symptoms from the MVA is a common event, often persisting for years after the accident. Myofascial pain, especially low back and pelvic, is typical. Piriformis syndrome, a form of sciatica due to spasm of one of the deep muscles of the buttock, is especially common, as it is in all patients with prior histories of sexual assault, rape, or incest. Gastrointestinal and menstrual symptoms frequently appear within a few months of the MVA. Sleep disturbance with dreams involving a state of helplessness are typical, and initial dreams of the MVA often give way to dreams of personal assault. Arousal, rage, and a sense of injustice for being injured in the MVA reflect the suppressed rage generated by the original sexual assault. This sense of outrage after rape is often suppressed by the shame and guilt that have been perpetuated by the rape myths of our society. Remarkably, many of these women had never had counseling for their rape, and many have discounted the effect of their rape on their lives prior to the MVA. Under these circumstances, addressing the repressed and latent arousal, rage, and fear related to their rape experience in the context of the emotional and physical pain caused by the MVA, affords an opportunity for real transformation.

MEDICAL TRAUMA

Anesthesia, Surgery, and Critical Medical Illness

Traumatic stress induced by exposure to our current allopathic and technological system in delivery of medical care has been addressed to a very limited degree in the standard medical literature. Because the concept of PTSD has been addressed for less than twenty years, emotional responses to medical interventions in the past have been considered predictable and justified, and usually of no consequence. If prolonged, these emotional responses were felt to fall into the category of neuroses, and often have been attributed to personality traits. Several factors in the development of modern medical techniques appear to be associated with the potential for traumatic stress. The introduction of ether anesthesia in the early twentieth century was a prelude to the rapid development of increasingly sophisticated surgical techniques, many of which were for the purpose of curing or relieving painful conditions, but most of which introduced the new dilemma of postsurgical pain. Anesthesia and surgery also introduced the cold, malodorous, and terrifying theater of the operating room, full of masked strangers, strange smells, and sounds into which one entered in a state of primitive and helpless nakedness.

Preoperative anxiety and panic have long been a significant concern to surgeons, from the standpoints of behavioral management, intraoperative complications, and postoperative outcomes. Fear of death, injury, postoperative pain, and even of helplessness and unconsciousness may be a source of preoperative anxiety.[58,59] Concerns about the effects of preoperative anxiety on both the physical and emotional outcomes of surgical procedures has led to the routine use of preoperative psychological support and sedation to minimize these risks.[58,60-62] Preoperative anxiety may be associated with rather remarkable psychophysiological changes related to sympathetic arousal that may be modified by preoperative medication.[63] The degree of sympathetic autonomic activation associated with marked preoperative anxiety is felt to increase the risk of thiopental induction by requiring a higher dose, thereby increasing the risk of circulatory collapse.[64]

Psychological and emotional responses to anesthesia and surgery have been documented, but the literature is remarkably sparse. Several studies have suggested that postoperative anxiety (A-State) is generally diminished compared to preoperative anxiety, and is unrelated to personality traits predisposing to anxiety (A-Trait).[65-67] This finding is in keeping with the logical explanation that preoperative anxiety may be heightened by fear of the unknown outcome and by the intrinsic threat of surgery, whereas postoperative anxiety is lessened by the gratifying awareness of having survived the ordeal.

Nevertheless, sleep disturbance and even nightmares have been reported fairly frequently in the postoperative days in surgical patients. Marked disruption of normal sleep patterns has been described in a group of patients during the early period of surgical convalescence.[68] A small group of twelve patients exhibited increased REM sleep, upsetting dreams, and nightmares beginning on the third postoperative night.[69] Delirium, sleep disturbance, and decreased REM sleep have been documented in patients after open-heart surgery, with no clear correlation with possible sources of hypoxia or ischemia.[70] Long-term emotional and psychological morbidity, however, is more difficult to interpret because the effect of the passage of time obscures the direct relationship of the patient's distress to the surgery itself.

A number of studies demonstrate the long-term psychological effects of surgery and potentially catastrophic illness. The major areas of study have been in the uniquely threatening diseases of cancer and myocardial infarction (MI), both of which carry a high risk of pain, disability, and death. Coronary artery disease is a predominantly male affliction, and by far the majority of coronary artery bypass grafts (CABG) are performed on men. Males have approximately one-third the likelihood of developing PTSD as a result of a given traumatic experience as females, and one therefore would expect the risk of developing PTSD in MI and CABG to be quite low. Studies, however, reflect an incidence of PTSD in 5 to 10 percent of males experiencing these events.[71,72] Symptoms in these cases primarily represented those of an intrusive variety and often persisted for over twelve months. Reexperiencing included both phobias of the illness itself with fears of recurrence, and intrusive memories and thoughts of particularly traumatic scenes from the acute hospital experience. Moderate to severe depression also occurred in another 8 percent.[72] It is clear that both the patient's awareness of suffering from a life-threatening disease, and an environment implying threat and helplessness contributed to the trauma.

One must consider in this context the physical environments of the operating room theater and intensive care unit (ICU), and what they represent to the terrified patient already burdened with the knowledge of potential impending mortality. For reasons of safety, hygiene, staff comfort, and efficiency, the environments are cold, bright, sterile, noisy, and clogged with frightening technological paraphernalia. Equipment emitting rhythmic beeping sounds measures the life forces of the patient, and every variation in sound implies potential disaster. At some point, CABG patients experience the terror of the sensation and sounds of a respirator pumping air into their lungs through an endotracheal tube, a condition of ultimate helplessness. Postoperative pain can be severe following a CABG procedure, and many patients report severe pain during the days following surgery despite narcotic analgesia. In this context, uncontrolled pain alone as an independent variable has been reported to be a cause of PTSD.[73]

On the other hand, these studies also show that the majority of the subjects did not suffer significant or long-term psychological distress. This is not altogether surprising considering the relative resistance to development of PTSD in males, but it again illustrates the fact that traumatic stress is not necessarily traumatizing in all individuals. These studies, however, did not investigate the potentially traumatic premorbid life experiences of the subjects. Based on experience with PTSD in combat veterans, MVAs, and other sources of trauma, prior life traumatic experiences should also play a role in traumatization associated with medical experiences.

Although studies addressing the development of PTSD in cancer patients are sparse, several shed light on the importance of prior life events and on the role of medical experiences themselves as a source of trauma. The significant occurrence of PTSD in cancer patients has begun to be explored primarily in the past decade.[74-79] The act of presenting a patient with even the possible diagnosis of a potentially fatal disease is consistent with a criteria-based stressor for PTSD based on the DSM-IV.[3] Following the diagnosis of cancer, patients are well known to vacillate between states of arousal/anxiety and dissociation/denial, a state comparable to the period following exposure to any overwhelming traumatic stress. This phenomenon had been documented in longitudinal studies of breast cancer patients that show that almost half of the patients diagnosed with cancer experienced high levels of intrusive anxiety prior to surgery, with significant reduction at six weeks after surgery.[78,79] One year after surgery, however, one-third still experienced insomnia due to intrusive thoughts or images from the illness, one-fifth experienced cancer-related nightmares, and over half experienced dissociative symptoms, especially numbness and feelings of unreality. Twelve percent still had criteria-based PTSD.[80] Not surprisingly, a number of premorbid factors were significantly predictive in development of symptoms of

PTSD in this population. Prior impaired psychosocial functioning, negative life events, health problems, and especially a personality trait characterized by high emotional reactivity, were all specifically noted to be risk factors for development of PTSD in this patient group.[80] The patient cohort in breast cancer is composed almost exclusively of females. This factor logically explains the increased incidence of symptoms of PTSD in this group, based on the increased risk of PTSD in females, probably due to their increased tendency to dissociate at the moment of traumatic stress. The fact that over half of the women experienced late symptoms of a dissociative nature is not surprising.

Although only a relatively small number of subjects developed criterion-based PTSD, the incidence and persistence of PTSD symptoms in these studies is remarkable. These statistics again remind us that the presentation of the diagnosis of serious or life-threatening disease to a patient alone may have serious and even long-term emotional consequences. The period of maximum arousal and anxiety symptoms in women with breast cancer occurred between the making of the diagnosis and informing the patient, and the immediate postoperative period. The immediate reassurance that the patients experienced having survived the surgery was sufficient to allay further anxiety and symptoms of PTSD in many patients. On the other hand, a great many went on to develop significant long-term symptoms of dissociation, sleep disturbance, anxiety attacks, and intrusive thoughts and memories, even though they perceived that they had been cured. The experience of fear, threat, and helplessness associated with the early period of their contact with the medical care system seems to have played a critical role in their subsequent emotional health.

Patients accessing the complex and highly technical medical system of diagnosis are by definition, exposed to perceived life threat in many instances. This frequently occurs in a relative state of helplessness. Physicians face the potential risk of contributing to the traumatization of their patients many times each day. The importance of effective and caring communication with their patients is generally poorly understood and frequently ignored when it comes to the concepts of healing, or conversely, traumatization. The remarkable power that physicians possess in determining the health of their patients solely through their personal contacts with them is addressed in books by holistic medical practitioners such as Larry Dossey[81] and

Bernie Siegel.[82] Caring communication is essentially ignored in the education of physicians, and yet, emotional attachment is probably the primary source of protection from being traumatized.

An intact social support network in the face of overwhelming traumatic stress will often shield the victim from the late symptoms of trauma. This particularly applies to children, whose emotionally and physically available caregivers are the primary factors in protecting them from traumatic stress.[83] In the case of serious illness, the physician may play the pivotal role in the patient's system of emotional and social support. Too often, physicians assume that patients cannot understand the complexity of the process by which they arrive at diagnostic and treatment decisions, and do not try to educate the patients and enlist them as partners in both the diagnostic and treatment processes. Telling a patient with back pain, "I really can't find anything seriously wrong, but I think we'd better get an MRI," means to the patient, "He's really more worried than he's willing to tell me; there must be something seriously wrong."

Approaching any diagnostic work-up for potentially serious disease will inevitably engender anxiety on the part of most patients. Enlisting them as informed and educated partners in the diagnostic process, however, lessens their sense of helplessness and loss of control, the primary factors that may predispose them to long-term emotional distress in the face of subsequent serious disease. This is especially important in the face of pressures to perform complex tests because of concerns about medical legal issues in our increasingly litigious medical system.

THE ROLE OF PAST TRAUMA

The previous breast cancer studies also illustrate the importance of being aware of the patient's legacy of traumatic experience when approaching diagnosis and treatment for serious disease. Premorbid life trauma, psychiatric or physical illness, or recent negative life events are all predictors of impaired emotional adjustment after serious illness. Identification of these risk factors in presurgical patients is basically ignored in current medical practice. Studies of PTSD and other psychiatric disorders implicate the patient's past emotional health in the development of these disorders. The medical and surgical literature has largely ignored the predictable emotional complications in these at-risk patients when confronted with diagnostic workup, surgery, or medical treatment for potentially life-threatening illness. The result is a large group of patients who develop delayed emotional symptoms, as well as a pattern of physical symptoms, especially chronic pain, which defy physiological and anatomical explanation. Failed back syndrome, persistent radicular pain attributed to "arachnoiditis," variations of reflex sympathetic dystrophy (RSD), and complex regional pain syndrome (CRPS) are examples of this dilemma.

Many of these chronic pain problems involve dissociation and somatization disorders, well-known late manifestations of PTSD. The tendency for victims of trauma, especially children, who have experienced dissociation to dissociate again when traumatized, is well documented (see Chapter 8). Such patients are also inordinately sensitive to threatening events that in other people might not be thought to represent trauma. The sterile and alien environment of the surgical theater may be sufficient in this patient population to trigger a dissociative reaction, leading to persistence of somatic manifestations of the presenting complaint despite anatomically corrective surgery. The analogy is similar to that of the previously traumatized victim of a trivial MVA who develops a full-blown whiplash syndrome. Patients with these specific problems, as well as myofascial pain, constitute the majority of referrals to chronic pain programs. The high incidence of past life trauma, especially child abuse, in the chronic pain population suggests that identification of patients with these risk factors before elective surgical intervention might help to avoid subsequent emotional morbidity, and the perpetuation of "nonphysiological" pain. Incorporation of preventative emotional and social support systems to deal with the helplessness and trauma of life-threatening disease, especially involving surgery, may be critical to ultimate healthy recovery in such patients.

AWARENESS DURING ANESTHESIA

Since the introduction of ether anesthesia by Morton in 1846, the occurrence of awareness during anesthesia has been well recognized and documented. Morton himself documented such a case during his career.[84] The resulting motor response of the patient awakening under anesthesia was usually sufficient to prompt the anesthetist to increase the depth of anesthesia, and shorten the period of the pain experience. With the introduction of curariform operative paralysis, however, patients lost the ability to respond to inadequate levels of anesthesia, and scientific reports of anesthetic awareness began to address the issue of posttraumatic neurosis in such patients.[85] Patient reports of awareness under anesthesia often addressed the overwhelming sense of helplessness that the patient experienced and the panic that it produced. Even in the absence of an experience of pain during the period of awareness, many patients developed symptoms of PTSD.[86] Typical symptoms in such a subject group include insomnia with sleep avoidance, flashbacks of paralysis and terror, flashbacks of pain with light sleep or with cues related to the operating theater. Panic or flashbacks with hospital-related cues, such as the color blue (scrub suits), medicinal smells, clinking silverware (surgical instruments), or hospital-related television shows are common.[87] In many cases, explicit recall of the events during the period of anesthetic awareness is remarkably clear and accurate, despite the fact that the anesthetic record did not reflect physiological changes that might give a clue to lightening of the depth of anesthesia.[88,89] Recall of negative comments by the operating team in these cases, especially when directed toward the patient, is noted to have particularly negative effects on emotional outcome. Clearly, explicit memory for events occurring during surgical anesthesia occurs in many cases of anesthetic awareness.

The role of explicit and implicit memory in trauma has been discussed (see Chapter 4). Explicit memory is verbal, semantic, conscious, and able to be elicited voluntarily. Implicit memory is not associated with conscious recall, but is represented by motor skills, conditioned responses, or emotions. Some studies suggest that implicit memory still may be involved in the processing and storage of information under anesthesia.[90] If so, those experiences associated with emotionally charged events, such as pain, paralysis, helplessness, or derogatory remarks while supposedly under anesthesia may be expected to contribute to intraoperative traumatization. The clinical features of memory in traumatic stress are characterized by their predominantly sensorimotor and emotional content, and by their relative lack of verbal or narrative content.[91] This fact emphasizes the role of implicit memory in the retention of memory for traumatic experiences. Even in the absence of explicit recall, the occurrence of unexplained postoperative emotional responses, unpredictable problems with pain control, or persistence of preoperative pain experiences despite successful surgery, might be due to the lightening of anesthesia during the surgery sufficient to imprint implicit memory for the experience.

The appearance of even partial symptoms of PTSD after a surgical procedure should raise concerns about a degree of lightening of anesthesia during the surgery sufficient to reproduce the emotional content of implicit memory through partial awareness. Since there is no accurate way to measure depth of anesthesia, the experience of partial awareness should not be ruled out even in the absence of explicit memory for events of the surgery. In addition, typical symptoms of PTSD may be obscured by the occurrence of dissociation or numbing following a traumatic anesthetic experience.

Awareness of events during a surgical procedure while paralyzed represents an ultimate expression of trauma in the face of helplessness, the prime condition for the development of PTSD. In the absence of any ability to exercise the fight/flight response, the inevitable response is the freeze or immobility response, the autonomic correlate of dissociation. Even if fragments of explicit memory for the events surrounding the awareness experience exist, they may be suppressed through dissociative amnesia. Reluctance by the patient to inform the surgeon or anesthesiologist of the episode of awareness has also been frequently documented, and may contribute to the physician's misunderstanding of supposedly unexplained postoperative distress.[84] Under such circumstances, emotional expression of the trauma may present in a delayed fashion in the form of somatization, dissociative symptoms, panic disorder, obsessive-compulsive disorder, or depression.[9] Physicians frequently attribute such postsurgical behaviors to the stress of the underlying illness or to premorbid maladaptive personality traits.

With these considerations in mind, prevention of morbidity from episodes of anesthetic awareness needs to be addressed through postoperative evaluation and debriefing. If clues to the experiencing of awareness during surgery are present, even if only in the form of unexplained somatic and emotional symptoms, counseling should be initiated. The goals of this counseling should include validation of the experience, assistance in recovering explicit memories of the event, and integration of these memories into a meaningful narrative. Exposure-based therapy may be necessary to desensitize the experience and place it into a benign perspective.

PEDIATRIC MEDICAL TRAUMA

Fetal and Neonatal Trauma

The idea that children might be traumatized by their contact with our system of medical care has been largely rejected for over a century. This concept was primarily based on the unfounded opinion by most physicians that infants could not process information, remember, learn, or for that matter feel pain, before myelination of frontal and limbic pathways has occurred. It was not until 1988 that the American Medical Association declared in a report on the most recent research that infants could feel pain. Before that date, many surgical procedures on infants were performed with only curariform paralysis without the benefit of general or local anesthesia.

Until about 1986, surgery for patent ductus arteriosus, involving insertion of arterial catheters and chest tubes, and thoracotomy with rib retraction, was performed in infants under only curariform paralysis. This traumatic experience involved one and one-half hours of exposure to complete helplessness and overwhelming pain without any concept of the effects of this trauma on the infant.[92] Chamberlain documents the case of a boy, born at twenty-nine weeks gestation, who underwent ventriculo-peritoneal shunting for hydrocephalus under curariform paralysis.[93] At fifteen, he was severely phobic about doctors, hospitals, medical procedures, and the sight of adhesive tape and bandages. He would not allow anyone to touch his head, neck, or abdomen, the site of his surgical incisions for the shunt operation. Clearly this neonate had experienced and processed the existential traumatic stress to which he had been exposed. Processing of traumatic memory takes place through implicit memory mechanisms and centers, many of which have achieved myelination during and even before the neonatal period. There is every reason to believe that perception and processing of pain experiences in the neonate are more than sufficient to induce the process of traumatization.

There is also ample evidence for early sentient interaction of new-born infants with their environment. Newborns and even fetuses in utero have been shown to be capable of classical habituation and con-ditioning.[94,95] Fetuses confronted with an amniocentesis needle invad-ing the uterus have been shown to exhibit fearful and defensive behavior.[96] Intrauterine needling of the fetus has been shown to elicit a full-blown stress-related increase in plasma cortisol and B-endorphin levels, with evidence that modulation of the stress response is slower than in the adult.[97] Fetuses can also learn to adapt their behavior to con-trol the environment. Through regulating the frequency of sucking on a nipple, an infant will learn to access his mother's voice when presented with a sequence of voices through headphones.[98] The evidence for learning in utero by the unborn fetus, in the pediatric intensive care unit by the premature infant and in the normal full-term newborn, is over-whelming.[99] The assumption that infants in all stages of development do not experience pain, do not register arousal with threat, and do not process a response to traumatic stress is clearly outdated and invalid. The risks of induction of traumatic stress in the medical management of the premature newborn and as-yet unborn fetus cannot be underesti-mated. When one takes a history of childhood trauma from a patient one usually addresses psychological, physical, and sexual abuse in the first decade. Little if anything in the PTSD literature addresses the ter-rible trauma to which premature infants are exposed, or the long-term behavioral and emotional sequelae of that trauma.

The other major threat facing the newborn infant is the modern day obstetrical theater. Infants born in the hospital face a cold, brilliantly bright, noisy environment associated with fetal monitoring probes in-serted in their scalp, metal forceps on their heads, the jabs of lancets in their heels, suction tubes in their noses, mouths, and tracheae, and caustic liquid instilled into their eyes. They also face separation and isolation from their mothers at the moment of birth, the most critical period for infant-maternal bonding, the period most important for early attunement. I personally viewed a "natural childbirth" video, developed for prenatal education classes, in which a mother gave birth to her infant in an unmedicated delivery with her husband in at-tendance. After the umbilical cord was cut, instead of placing the baby on her mother's breast, the nurse took the infant to a bassinet, where she began to perform vigorous nasotracheal suction. The infant exhibited a vigorous Moro (startle) reflex, but after two or three assaultive suction sequences, the infant became limp and unresponsive. When the infant was finally placed on the mother's breast, it remained limp and immobile, locked into its very first freeze response in the face of needless and brutal traumatization by a supposed caregiver.

The current medical philosophy of birth appears to be driven by the pervasive fear of injury to the newborn infant that, unfortunately, is partly based on medicolegal concerns, as well as the increasing worship of the technology of medicine. Although there is overwhelming evidence that fetal monitoring and a higher rate of cesarean sections has not lessened fetal mortality or morbidity, the standard use of these invasive procedures has now been established as a benchmark for obstetrical care. Fetal morbidity in the absence of these procedures is considered a red flag for litigation.

Birth is an inherently natural process. It provides the earliest opportunity for enhancement of infant brain development required to provide resiliency in the face of threat through early maternal bonding. The brain at this stage of life is not at its most adaptable state; it is rather at its most vulnerable. Exposing the newborn to traumatic stress through thoughtless invasive and painful medical procedures is senseless and dangerous. Many child psychologists feel that the roots of societal violence, at least in part, relate to birth trauma.[93] A large study of 4,200 consecutive births revealed that the combination of birth complications and maternal separation were powerful predictors of violent crimes in later life.[100]

Male infant circumcision, still often performed without anesthesia, continues to be one of the most blindly accepted but inherently traumatic experiences of the neonate. While the male newborn is immobilized by wrapping it in a sheet, the penis is swabbed with alcohol to induce an erection, a clamp is placed over the penile foreskin and painfully tightened, and the foreskin excised in a circular fashion with a scalpel. The procedure is so "simple" that most medical students, including myself, have been allowed to perform it. The infant will be observed to cry bitterly, often exhibit a series of Moro reflexes, and then lapse into immobility. Only recently have physicians begun to advocate local anesthesia when performing circumcisions. Recent studies reveal that circumcised boys show significantly more severe emotional response to vaccination injections at ages four and six months than boys who have not been circumcised.[101] Over 60 percent of American male infants continue to be circumcised.[102] In

March 1999, the American Academy of Pediatrics established a policy recommending that newborn males receive pain relief for circumcision, admitting that the pain experienced by infants at circumcision could have long-lasting side effects.[102]

CHILDHOOD MEDICAL TRAUMA

Both neonatal and pediatric stress responses, measured by the release of catabolic stress hormones, are significant in anesthesia and surgical settings and are relatively greater in magnitude than adult responses to similar medical procedures.[103] The brains of young children, therefore, regulate arousal less efficiently than adults, and are more susceptible to traumatization. Not surprisingly, emotional and behavioral problems have been reported often in children subjected to anesthesia and surgery. The procedure studied the most is childhood tonsillectomy. As always, the measures used to assess such responses affect interpretation of the outcomes. In general, phobic and disruptive behaviors seem to be the most common, and appear to be time limited and reduced by presurgical emotional support.[104] Responses indicating traumatization are by no means universal, but when present, may be quite dramatic.

Perhaps the most potent evidence lies in the stories themselves, in this case involving a number of my own medical colleagues who have undergone ether anesthesia and tonsillectomy in their first decade. One recalls that for many years thereafter, he could not spontaneously yawn without feeling panic and stifling the yawn. He recalls the operating room nurse encouraging him to inhale deeply during ether induction, an act that for years he found threatening when it involved yawning. Another colleague who underwent five experiences of ether anesthesia before the age of eleven had a phobia of falling asleep throughout his childhood, primarily due to a fear of being unconscious. He also had a morbid childhood phobia of the smell of ether and other volatile chemicals. His pursuit of the medical profession can only be attributed to traumatic reenactment. Many of us in the medical profession recall being allowed to perform ether anesthesia induction on children for tonsillectomy under the supervision of an anesthetist. The event is characterized by wrapping the child in a sheet while an orderly forcibly holds the child down to the gurney. A gauze-covered metal cone is clamped over the child's nose and mouth, and ether is dripped from a can onto the gauze while the child screams and thrashes. During the surgery, the mask must be removed for the surgical procedure itself, as well as for suctioning, and then placed back on the face to deepen anesthesia when the child begins to gag and cough due to the secretions and blood. The scene can only be described as barbaric, and the child exposed to it no doubt experiences the same horror.

The practice of immobilizing children by wrapping them in a sheet and isolating them from their mother when performing simple emergency room suturing for routine lacerations has all of the elements of threat and helplessness required to induce traumatic stress. One patient described the injection of local anesthetic for a scalp laceration as terrifying, and still recalls the certainty that the doctor was injecting his brain, and that he was going to die. Another child who was separated from her mother for essentially the same procedure, demonstrated anger and rejection of her mother, and acting-out behavior for months thereafter.

Unfortunately, more detailed or controlled studies of the effects of our technological system of medicine on children are not available at this time. Anecdotal medicine is uniformly rejected as a means of arriving at meaningful scientific conclusions, and for good reason. Using the words, "in my experience," to justify a medical conclusion merits immediate skepticism; yet, catastrophic complications of medical procedures also merit immediate attempts to correct the fallacies in those procedures. Applying the concepts of traumatic stress to many current medical practices, reviewing the data from analogous sources of trauma in our society, and recognizing the results of that trauma should compel us to reassess some of our current standards of treatment for our patients, especially our children and infants. Anecdotal experience in medical practice does suggest that traumatization with all of the features discussed previously occurs with shocking frequency, and undoubtedly, contributes significantly to the load of life trauma that ultimately may have devastating long-term effects on the individual.

CONCLUSION

I have only touched on the numerous sources of trauma in our world and society, neglecting entirely issues of torture, imprisonment, genocide, civilian experiences in war, and natural disasters to name but a few. I have previously addressed the role of motor vehicle accidents as a relatively unappreciated source of cultural trauma. I have also emphasized what I perceive to be a generally neglected source of trauma, our current system of medicine, because I am familiar with it, both as a childhood patient and a practitioner. I also see its influence on patients who suffer from chronic pain, often not because of an injury but because of the tests and procedures used to diagnose and treat the pain. Trauma will always be with us. Our bodies are designed to deal with it as an inevitable life occurrence. It certainly behooves us as the caregivers and healers who attempt to lessen the ravages of unresolved trauma not to contribute to its effects through procedures, institutions, traditions, and behaviors that unknowingly serve to initiate or perpetuate trauma.

Chapter 10

Trauma Therapy:
Future Directions

Marge, at fifty, awoke daily with the stiffened tissues and dragging fatigue of the fibromyalgia patient. She had been disabled for a decade by the pain, exhaustion, and intrusive and muddled thoughts associated with this puzzling condition, and despaired of any hope of recovery. I saw her for a friend, one of the therapists in town who practiced Somatic Experiencing, and was not optimistic about her chances for healing with trauma therapy, since she clearly was markedly dissociated from normal perception of her body and had no clear-cut history of inordinate life trauma. Nevertheless, at his encouragement we enrolled her in pool therapy utilizing Watsu, a warm water-based form of shiatsu massage, in this case also incorporating body tracking of the "felt sense," part of the technique of somatic experiencing. With Marge's first exposure to this technique, she had a severe dissociative episode, in the form of a pseudoseizure. Using great caution, my friend and the Watsu therapist continued to treat her, stopping the pool therapy at the first sign of dissociation, and immediately taking her to a small room where she was allowed to recover, wrapped in blankets and resourced by the therapist. Invariably Marge would go through a stereotyped pattern of body trembling and deep breathing until she recovered, a process often taking over an hour.

After several months of cautious weekly treatment, she began to show strange gulping and gasping behavior as part of her recovery from her Watsu sessions. For the first time, she recalled that her mother had told her about her very traumatic birth, with strangulation by the umbilical cord requiring intubation and assisted respiration for over twenty-four hours. With the appearance of this unusual respiratory response to the Watsu sessions, her morning pain began to clear, her sleep became restorative, and her sense of cognitive slowing cleared. She continues to manifest slow but remarkable remission of symptoms of fibromyalgia, but also remains extremely vulnerable to recurrence of symptoms with any life stress.

* * *

My goal in this chapter is to integrate existing opinions and data on the most accepted methods of therapy for PTSD into an approach to therapy based on somatic concepts of trauma. I strongly feel that new models of somatically based treatment for trauma need to be explored and tested in the light of emerging data concerning the psychophysiological basis for PTSD, and the theories presented in this book. With this understanding in mind, I beg the forbearance of my psychology and psychiatry colleagues, and hope that the ideas presented may be applicable to some of their treatment paradigms.

With the addition to the DSM-III in 1980 of post-traumatic stress disorder as a diagnosis distinct from other anxiety-based disorders,[1] increasing attention has been given to specific treatment models for this common problem. Group therapy involving trauma victims has been a mainstay of treatment since combat-related trauma was again brought to the world's attention after World War II.[2] The impetus to explore treatment models was again revived by the Vietnam War experience, and by the designation of PTSD as a unique condition. Based on these experiences, enhancement of interpersonal connections through family and social support systems, including those involving fellow victims of trauma, has become a central thesis for therapeutic management of PTSD. This approach, together with other forms of cognitive therapy, falls under the category of resourcing the victim's own self-regulatory mechanisms for dealing with the intrusion of painful emotional and physical symptoms. Although limited in scope, these therapies provide a useful start to the process of traumatic healing.

COUNSELING
AND VERBAL/COGNITIVE THERAPY

Memory mechanisms in trauma guarantee that the access to these memories and their meanings in a verbal context may be difficult or impossible. As we have noted in Chapter 4, traumatic memories tend to be stored in an emotional or somatic context, and the victim simply may not be able to place them in a verbal context. Alexithymia, the inability to adequately express emotions or body sensations in words, undoubtedly relates to this problem. A review in Chapter 11 of personal case studies in trauma from my own practice documents a class of patients presenting with bizarre disorders of stuttering, speech blockage, and impairment of immediate verbal processing, clearly on a dissociative basis. Although from a psychiatric standpoint, dissociation is felt to be a fragmentation of conscious awareness, I have attempted to present dissociation as a measurable physiological event, both at the level of the central nervous system and at the dissociated end organ (see Chapter 8).

In this light, a regional physiological basis for these verbal impairments in trauma victims, as well as for alexithymia, may well exist based on recent positron emission tomography (PET) findings. Impairment of verbal expression in trauma may have its roots in reflex inhibition of metabolic function in portions of the left cerebral hemisphere, especially Broca's area.[3] References to "speechless terror," and other metaphorical analogies reflect the well-recognized inhibition of verbal functions in trauma. Cognitive therapy involving verbal interaction, insight, and interpretation under these conditions of impairment of verbal expression would be predictably difficult. This dilemma is in keeping with the conclusions of many trauma specialists that "talking about the trauma" is rarely sufficient to dissipate the self-perpetuating trauma cycle.[4]

Nevertheless, verbal cognitively based therapy appears to play an important part in initiating the therapeutic process in trauma. The role of the therapist in providing guidance, interpretation, and education through verbal interaction is critical, especially early in the traumatic response. Stabilization through anxiety control skills and identification of the meaning of somatic sensations that represent uncomfortable feeling states, enable the patient to cope with self-perpetuating states of arousal. Encouraging trauma victims to verbalize these somatic sensations may allow them to access and integrate intense feeling states into conscious awareness. Hopefully, doing so may help to diminish the dissociation that contributes to substitution of somatic discomfort for intense emotions. Since access to the underlying hyperarousal and anxiety associated with trauma is painful, the presence of the therapist is important in providing a supportive environment for the process. Patients with PTSD suffer from sensitivity to any arousal stimulus. Elicitation of their fight/flight response has become generalized to a wide variety of nonspecific environmental trauma-related cues, in addition to nonspecific sources of arousal. As a result, a trusting environment is extremely important for trauma patients, based to a considerable extent on their predictably increased sensitivity to the nuances of the therapist's behavior and demeanor. Even the facial characteristics or behavioral quirks of the therapist may remind patients of threatening past experiences or perpetrators of their trauma. As a result, great care must be taken to provide an environment of safety and trust to allow the patient to access painful and arousing memories in a form that is bearable and in a setting that is perceived as safe. Bringing these memories and feelings into consciousness, and providing a narrative verbal format for the experience, appears to be necessary to begin the process of integrating the memories into conscious experience, and presumably to inhibit the patient's cue-related arousal recycling. By learning to apply words to these terrible feelings and memories, the patient may begin to attain skills in containing and to some extent controlling them, and in relegating them to past experience rather than to an ongoing traumatic experience.[5]

Patient education is also an important therapeutic goal. Most patients can understand complexities of psychophysiological concepts that might surprise many therapists. Providing a logical cognitive format for the patient's somatic and emotional symptoms serves several important functions. Most patients with symptoms characteristic of somatization and affect dysregulation have been labeled and devalued by their medical providers because they are felt to show symptom magnification, psychosomatic symptoms, or behavior indicating secondary gain. Dismissal or approbation by the very people upon whom trauma victims are dependent for support and care enhances and perpetuates the physiological trauma cycle. The pain and suffering that they experience with perceived rejection is greatly enhanced by their intrinsic vulnerability, and as real to them as acute surgical pain.

Most of my traumatized MVA patients experience a period of marked deterioration of both somatic and emotional symptoms when their insurance company begins to question provider reimbursement or begins the first round of independent medical examinations, and when their legal case becomes active. Their response is usually one of helpless rage, self-doubt, and a sense of devaluation. This process continues to reinforce their state of helplessness, the very basis for their trauma. Under this environment of renewed threat, these patients often experience a recurrence of the entire constellation of physical, cognitive, and emotional symptoms of whiplash.

Detailed education and information about the very valid physiological basis for their physical and emotional symptoms is empowering and restores the sense of control needed for their recovery. Providing words for the meaning of these frightening sensations begins the process of integrating them into a narrative format and a logical cognitive construct. Knowledge and enlightenment in this environment are critical to reestablishing a sense of validity, and restoring a sense of self in the trauma victim.

Enlightenment through education, however, attacks only one facet of the trauma edifice. Knowledge allows the patient to deal with the unbidden and recurrent symptoms of trauma at a higher level, to facilitate interpretation and understanding, and thereby to help the patient achieve some degree of control over painful sensations or memories when they arise. Knowledge does not alter the basic kindled cycle of arousal, recall, muscle bracing, and autonomic cycling that perpetuates trauma. Ultimately, one must gain access to the insidious conditioned trauma response from a physiological and unconscious reflexive approach in order to extinguish, desensitize, inhibit, or quench it. Since such a therapeutic process is likely to present substantial risks of flooding and retraumatization, cognitive resourcing and empowerment is clearly indicated. Early limited cognitive therapy may, therefore, play an important role in preparing the patient for other, more confrontational, techniques such as exposure or desensitization.

EXPOSURE AND DESENSITIZATION TECHNIQUES

In an attempt to change and extinguish many of the intrusive symptoms of PTSD, more confrontational and invasive techniques of therapy have evolved. The technique with the best documentation is cognitive-behavioral therapy, a method designed to change the implications or meaning of intrusive symptoms. The various techniques under this category share, to some extent, the process of extinction of a conditioned response by eliciting the response (memory, emotion) in an environment that does not contain a trigger (cues, threat) for that response. The meaning of the response in relation to the basic survival instinct is changed and diminished as exposure to the response occurs repeatedly in a benign environment. As a result, habituation through repeated exposure progressively diminishes the fear/arousal response in PTSD. Such techniques as imaginal exposure and systematic desensitization involve guided reexperiencing of traumatic memories and images in a controlled therapeutic setting.

Numerous studies suggest that these techniques have a substantial therapeutic effect on reducing intrusive and cue-related arousal symptoms in PTSD.[6-9] Flooding, however, may carry significant risk. Intense arousal and reexperiencing may duplicate the original traumatic experience, and without a concomitant internal and external environment that incorporates a sense of safety and empowerment, the victim may move immediately into the freeze response. Severe dissociative reactions and enduring aversive psychological symptoms may complicate therapeutic techniques incorporating flooding.[10] In addition, most studies document that the primary PTSD symptoms that benefit from exposure techniques are those involving arousal, fear, and traumatic reexperiencing. Late symptoms of avoidance, dissociation, somatization, and depression may be less responsive to cognitive-behavioral techniques.

Many of the clinical studies in these techniques also suffer from methodological problems, often related to standard outcome measures. Also, the spectrum of expression of symptoms in PTSD varies greatly, with wide variation in manifestation of symptoms of arousal and avoidance. Gender differences in response to trauma play a significant role in efficacy of various techniques, as might be expected. The nature of the traumatic stress and the context of the environment in which it occurred predictably produce variations in the clinical manifestations of the resulting traumatic symptoms. Studies comparing the effectiveness of therapy for PTSD in female assault victims are, therefore, likely to show significantly different outcomes than similar therapy in Vietnam War veterans, both because of gender differences and the nature of the traumatic experience. By themselves, these studies do not necessarily reflect the efficacy of a technique useful in one population but not useful in another. Indeed, studies of Vietnam veterans in general show resistance to many therapeutic techniques, including pharmacotherapy, a finding that has been attributed at least in part to the association of guilt with the traumatic experience.[11]

Adverse responses to exposure techniques by Vietnam veterans have raised concerns that reinforcement of guilt in exposure techniques might substantiate rather than desensitize arousal and anxiety. Based on these concerns, Rothbaum and Foa advocate developing techniques for guilt reduction because of its prevalence in PTSD in general.[12] Meanwhile they recommend the use of exposure-based therapy for arousal-related symptoms, and cognitive techniques for issues related to guilt.

Several mechanisms have been proposed to account for the apparent efficacy of exposure-based therapies for PTSD.[13] Habituation through repetitive exposure to the precipitating internal or external cue for the traumatic response might lessen the arousal response and correct the notion that anxiety is inevitable unless avoidance or dissociation is activated. Second, deliberate confrontation with the traumatic memories blocks or inhibits negative reinforcement associated with the repetitive arousal/avoidance cycle. Third, repeatedly reexperiencing the traumatic experience through confrontation or memory in a safe and supportive setting incorporates the message of safety into the traumatic memory, helping the patient to realize that the memory itself is not dangerous. Fourth, focusing intently on the traumatic memory or cue for a prolonged period of time separates it from the nontraumatic portion of the patient's existence, thereby reducing the patient's tendency to generalize the trauma to any arousal cue. Fifth, imaginal reexperiencing assists the patient in restructuring the meaning of traumatic memories from representing states of helplessness and incompetence to states of mastery and control. Finally, repeated exposure to traumatic memories allows patients to focus on those portions of the experience that reflect negatively on themselves, and to modify those perceptions into a positive model.[13]

Techniques directed toward anxiety management have also been employed extensively in PTSD treatment. These techniques are designed to develop coping skills in lessening arousal and anxiety, and generally involve body-training exercises, often supplemented with biofeedback. Examples include deep muscle relaxation, breathing exercises, thought stopping, cognitive restructuring, covert modeling, and stress inoculation. All of these techniques employ active intervention by the patient in diminishing painful somatic or emotional symptoms through learned techniques of self-regulation designed to control or diminish that part of the trauma cycle involving arousal. They do not address symptoms of avoidance and dissociation. Indeed, it is theoretically possible that a number of these techniques might enhance dissociative tendencies as a means of achieving relief from arousal symptoms, since the only objective measures for success are based on reduction of measures or symptoms of physiological arousal. It is no surprise that these techniques in general do show improvement in arousal symptoms after treatment, lasting as long as six months in cases, but studies testing them contain methodological flaws, including lack of confirmation of PTSD diagnostic criteria. Nevertheless, studies combining anxiety management and exposure techniques seem to show that a combination of these approaches might present the best clinically tested treatment for chronic PTSD.[12]

SOMATICALLY BASED THERAPIES

A varied, eclectic, largely unproven but intriguing body of somatically based trauma therapies has emerged in the past decade, driven by a number of factors. These include the relative resistance in trauma victims to treatment of PTSD, the frustrating inadequacies of many psychological treatment models, the recognition of the psychophysiological base for PTSD, and the emergence of so-called mind/body and alternative medicine. In addition, many of the treatment methods that have been used in the past focus extensively on reduction in symptoms of arousal, the most obvious sources of distress in this patient population. These techniques do not, however, appear to have a consistently measurable effect on reduction of avoidance or dissociation in published studies. In the model of PTSD and dissociation presented here, this relative deficiency represents a critical flaw in current accepted treatment methods for PTSD.

Some of the somatically based therapies are founded on solid theoretical but unproven physiological models of trauma and traumatization. Some involve stereotyped visual, auditory, tactile, or vestibular stimulation in a variety of settings with or without imaging of past traumatic events. Some involve repetitive verbal incantations, generally involving self-realization and empowerment, sometimes associated with tapping of acupuncture meridian points. A number involve the practice of kinesiology, a technique also related to concepts of Eastern medicine, acupuncture meridians, and the flow of "energy" within the body. Many have a revelatory therapeutic experience with one of their patients by the founder of the technique, often on a serendipitous basis. This sentient event is subsequently followed by a post hoc experiential definition and refinement of the practice of the technique, and the development of a theoretical physiological rationale for its effect. Theories explaining the mechanisms for the therapeutic effect are often couched in a vocabulary unique to the technique itself. Finally, a training workshop format with accreditation criteria for practitioners is established. Of these techniques, only Eye Movement Desensitization and Reprocessing (EMDR) has been subjected to significant scientific scrutiny using controlled trials.

The clinical appeal of these therapies relates to their apparent relative simplicity, and the quick results that are often reported, especially in clearing phobic and arousal symptoms. Considering the resistance to therapy of chronic PTSD, the enthusiastic response of many psychotherapists to these techniques is not surprising. The eclectic and largely unexplained rationale for effectiveness of these techniques and the skepticism of the behavioral science academic community is also not surprising. Most have not been exposed to appropriate rigorous scientific scrutiny. Nevertheless, the most publicized and studied of these techniques, EMDR, is clearly beginning to make inroads into the realm of acceptance as a valid treatment model for PTSD.

I have chosen to highlight and discuss these techniques, not because I feel that they necessarily represent the template for future treatment models for PTSD. Rather, I feel that they are intriguing because they represent a somatically based reflexive approach to a condition that is characterized by the predominantly unconscious perpetuation of conditioned and reflexive neural responses. Decades of treatment techniques for PTSD that are based on cognitive intent have shown consistently positive results in subpopulations of PTSD victims. However, they have also failed to break the underlying kindled response and to dispel the dominance of dissociation in many patients.

Although individual somatically based reflexive techniques may conceivably lead to a therapeutic dead end, I think that it is likely that components of these techniques may provide pathways to resolution of the physiological manifestations of trauma that remain a barrier to many of the existing accepted trauma therapies.

EYE MOVEMENT DESENSITIZATION
AND REPROCESSING

In 1989, Shapiro discovered quite by chance that rapidly moving one's eyes while thinking of arousal-based memory lessened the anxiety associated with that memory for a prolonged time. The discovery was made as part of a personal experience, and as a psychotherapist, she began to apply a technique that she developed from this experience on her patients with PTSD.[14] Eye Movement Desensitization (EMD), as she called it, entailed the identification of a traumatic memory by the patient associated with the expression of a personal "negative cognition" ("I am shameful"), followed and replaced by a "positive cognition" ("I am honorable"). The therapist would then pass her fingers back and forth in front of the patient's face for ten to twelve cycles while the patient followed them visually and concentrated on the traumatic memory. Following each trial, the therapist would assess the status of the patient's distress in relationship to the memory, and the degree of incorporation of the positive cognition. In her 1989 early report, Shapiro claimed remarkable clearing of the negative affective component of the traumatic memory in all of her PTSD patients. As she developed the theoretical basis for her technique, she added the term "reprocessing" to its name (EMDR) based on her conclusion that the technique enhanced the speed of information processing and facilitated transformation within the traumatic memory.

The results of anecdotal studies documenting the apparent efficacy of EMDR began to spread throughout the psychotherapeutic community and hundreds of therapists have received training in the technique through workshops developed by Shapiro. The eclectic nature of the technique predictably has raised skepticism within the same community as well. Early studies attempting to validate the technique were primarily outcome studies using standardized measures of symptoms and the state of distress before and after treatment. Even large studies suggest universal short-term improvement in symptoms of hyperarousal, intrusion, and avoidance.[15] Follow-up studies suggest good retention of therapeutic benefits.[16] On the other hand, uncontrolled studies have been challenged with the assertion that results could well have been based solely on the placebo effect associated with patient contact, and that outcome studies do nothing to validate the unique therapeutic benefit of the eye movement process itself.

Controlled studies have now been done in EMDR, and give a mixed picture regarding patient benefit and validation of the technique. Several studies have been done comparing EMDR with nontreatment wait list patients with PTSD. Although comparison with a nontreatment group of patients does not negate the placebo effect, EMDR clearly appears to produce substantially more improvement than no treatment over a similar period of time.[16,17] Comparison of EMDR to a number of techniques that have not been validated in PTSD (relaxation, biofeedback, active listening, image habituation) suggests that there is either no difference between techniques[18] nor superiority of EMDR.[19,20] Only one randomized and controlled study compares EMDR with a validated treatment technique for PTSD. In comparison with cognitive-behavioral therapy (CBT), this study showed that EMDR was less effective than CBT in reducing PTSD symptoms, both statistically and clinically, and that this disparity was actually more evident at a three-month follow-up.[21]

Another concern raised about the specific technique of EMDR questions the relative roles of the eye movements themselves, the traumatic memory imagery, and the use of negative and positive cognitive processes. Shapiro has steadfastly maintained that the eye movements themselves remain the core element of the technique.[14] As a result, researchers have attempted to "dismantle" the various components of EMDR in an attempt to discover the salient therapeutic elements. The results have been both startling and confusing. One study suggested that eye movements alone without the cognitive elements of EMDR produced therapeutic benefits comparable to those achieved by the standard treatment protocol.[22] Another study using alternate tapping on left and right fingers of the subject showed comparable clinical efficacy, but less change in measures of autonomic arousal.[23] A third demonstrated no difference between using the EMDR protocol with eye movement or with the eyes fixed, although, compared to a past study by these investigators, EMDR was at least as effective as imaginal flooding.[24] Although these studies cast doubt on the critical nature of the eye movement component of EMDR as maintained by Shapiro, they by no means disprove the efficacy of the entire protocol in comparison to other generally accepted techniques.

Speculation about the physiological mode of action of such therapeutic modalities proves nothing, but it provides the basis for studies designed to validate it, to dissect its therapeutic elements, and to apply that knowledge to devising ancillary treatments. Shapiro presents the hypothesis that the traumatic event leading to the associated memory is isolated and static because it has never been integrated or processed into an adaptive level. EMDR is physiologically designed to allow that reprocessing to take place.[25] As we have noted, positron emission tomography (PET) studies in arousal activation in PTSD patients suggest a significant lack of physiological coherence between the cerebral hemispheres in patients with PTSD. Several studies using quantitative EEG (QEEG), and single photon emission computerized tomography (SPECT), also support this concept of impairment of cerebral hemispheric synchronicity in PTSD, and show preliminary evidence for integration and reactivation of metabolically inhibited regions in the left hemisphere by relatively brief treatment with EMDR.[26,27] Others have noted that alternate finger tapping and auditory stimuli seem to have an equivalent effect in diminishing symptoms of arousal in PTSD.[28]

All of these somatic techniques have the production of rhythmic alternating bilateral cerebral hemispheric stimulation in common. This has led several authors to suggest that this integrative effect on cerebral function may help to restore cortical control of sensitized and kindled limbic and brainstem structures. This process might occur from the top down through facilitation of cortical control of limbic structures,[26,27] or from the bottom up, through down-regulation of limbic and brainstem nuclei.[28]

"Positive cognition" in EMDR and a number of other techniques also appear to play an independent and important role in the therapeutic process. As noted, positive thinking may produce symptomatic improvement by itself. Activation of inhibited left hemispheric speech and language centers through repetitive verbalization, especially of a phrase with a positive emotional valence, might well facilitate bilateral cerebral coherence and integration, and enhance the effects of the accompanying somatic exercise. All of these hypotheses, of course, are speculative at this time. They do, however, point the way to avenues of investigation, both of the validity of EMDR and for the development of similar therapeutic techniques to achieve similar physiological goals. One of the most exciting aspects of this process is the attempt to view and conceptualize trauma therapy in terms of its brain pathophysiology and to approach that physiology as a benchmark for treatment. Another is the recognition that the body plays a critical role in the manifestation and perpetuation of trauma, and may be a potent avenue for accessing and dissipating the core physiology of the traumatic reflex.

SOMATIC EXPERIENCING

The technique of Somatic Experiencing developed by Levine[29] for the treatment of trauma is what led me to my interest in PTSD and, ultimately, to this book. Somatic Experiencing has had far less application than EMDR, and has not been subjected to scientific scrutiny. SE is unique and intriguing in that it does not rely on specific cognitive elements to achieve its effects. Levine's theory of trauma uses the animal model of the fight/flight/freeze response in the wild. He notes that when animals can no longer escape a predator, they enter a freeze or immobility state, during which the high-level metabolic and neurochemical energy of the flight response continues despite the immobility of the freeze response. If the animal survives, the stored energy is dissipated through various stereotyped somatic and autonomic responses, including trembling, perspiring, and deep breathing. Human beings tend not to dissipate this energy, possibly through acculturated social restraint or neocortical inhibition, resulting in the storage of arousal-based energy. This phenomenon then leads to the complex physiological process of PTSD. Of interest is the fact that Levine links the late somatic manifestations and symptoms of trauma to this process, incorporating somatization, denial, affect dysregulation, and depression into the entire trauma response.

Although Levine addresses the process of traumatic memory in the generation of symptoms, he emphasizes the role of procedural or implicit memory in the storage of traumatic energy, and incorporates explicit cognitive processes to a limited extent in his therapy. He uses the "felt sense" to pursue and access the trauma response. Levine describes this somatic state of being primarily by example rather than by specific definition. A working definition of the felt sense might be the sum total of all sensations from all sense organs, both conscious and subliminal, at any given moment.

Since the brain rapidly filters and discards unnecessary sensory input, much of the felt sense is unconscious until one concentrates purposely on feeling the subtleties of somatic awareness. SE involves exploration of these sensations by the patient under the guidance of a therapist trained in the technique. When patients with PTSD or its late manifestations access the felt sense, they will eventually arrive at awareness of subtle somatic sensations that represent somasthetic procedural memory for a traumatic experience. The patients will then be guided initially to experience the sensation more intensely, and then to retreat to a previously established imaginary "safe place" as they begin to experience arousal triggered by the developing link to the limbic portion of that memory. By titrating in and out of this "trauma vortex" with the guidance of the therapist, the patient will eventually undergo the stereotyped motor and autonomic "discharge" of traumatic energy typified in animals emerging from the freeze response. This response is remarkably stereotyped in human subjects, suggesting a common physiological response. It will usually involve an involuntary motor response that often reflects the movement patterns experienced in a protective fashion during the traumatic event. "Completion" of that movement is felt to be an important event in dissipation of the procedural memory for the trauma and its link to arousal.

SE presents another interesting approach to what we know about the neurophysiology of trauma. Its primary appeal may lie in its noncognitive approach to what is primarily a brainstem and limbic phenomenon. Accessing and eliciting a motor response linked to a kindled limbic event in a benign environment, and completing the response successfully, could exert a powerful effect on down-regulating these sensitized and kindled subcortical circuits. Levine believes that one need not access explicit memory for the core traumatic event for SE to successfully discharge the traumatic energy, although at times it may be a useful adjunct to facilitating the technique. The risk of flooding, including the recovery of traumatic amnestic events, is moderate, hence the use of titration by the therapist. In general, SE appears to provide remarkable control of the therapeutic process.

My clinical impression based on experience with several hundred patients treated with both SE and EMDR is that SE tends to result in resolution of dissociative traits and behaviors more effectively than many techniques. I am also extremely impressed with the safety and efficacy of SE in the common problem of the traumatized patient with chronic pain. Myofascial pain is ubiquitous in the chronic pain population, and extremely resistant to treatment. Based on my theory that myofascial pain reflects procedural memory for regional muscular bracing patterns experienced at the moment of a life-threatening event, one might suspect that uncoupling of that memory from associated kindled arousal might mitigate the pain. This concept is in keeping with the theoretical basis for SE, and indeed, I have found in many patients that chronic pain, especially myofascial pain, may show striking improvement as part of the SE therapeutic process. Obviously SE needs to be scrutinized through controlled outcome and physiological studies before any conclusions regarding specific aspects of its efficacy can be validated.

THE "POWER THERAPIES"

In a widely criticized, and in fact at times condemned, study done in 1995 at Florida State University, Charles Figley gathered together founders and practitioners of a group of eclectic, controversial, but widely used, trauma therapies. The purpose of the meeting was to have the founder of each technique present its basic tenets to the attendees, and to perform an admittedly crude experiment to compare these techniques and to study their "active ingredients."[32] These therapies have come to be known in some circles as the "power therapies."

The designation of the therapies to be studied was derived from an Internet-based survey sent to about 10,000 practitioners of trauma therapy requesting opinions about methods of treatment for PTSD that were basically quick, easy, and effective based on the endorsement of at least 300 therapists. The results of the survey yielded four techniques judged by Figley and his group to represent the most widely used and effective tools based on the combined opinions of the respondents. These four techniques included the previously discussed Eye Movement Desensitization and Reprocessing (EMDR), as well as Visual/Kinesthetic Disassociation (VKD), Traumatic Incident Reduction (TIR), and Thought Field Therapy (TFT). All of these techniques represented empirically based methods that, except for EMDR, had not received scientific scrutiny. The therapies were presented and studied at the meeting at Florida State University and the results were discussed. The patient subjects were gleaned from the population of the Tallahassee, Florida, area by radio, newspaper articles, and word of mouth, and were admitted to the project based on a history of trauma or phobia without concern for strict diagnostic criteria for PTSD. The random assignment of patients to each one of the four therapies broke down, however, and all research participants expressed concern about the study's methodology.

The primary measure of treatment success was the Subjective Unit of Distress Scale (SUDS), a self-reported symptom scale measured from 1 to 10 based on the severity of symptoms of distress. Despite all of the problems with the design and administration of the test, all techniques demonstrated significant SUDS reduction that persisted after six months in most participants, but with some rebound in distress scales at six months within all of the techniques. The small number of patients studied in each technique, and the problems with methodology, however, prevented any statistically significant conclusions from being drawn.

VKD is based on the premise that the patient with PTSD is locked into a memory of the trauma associated with its negative feeling state.[30] The goal of treatment is to disassociate the memory from the negative emotion. This is achieved through the process of the therapist guiding the patient to visualize the traumatic event in the third person as if watching a movie. The memory/movie is then run from back to front, or front to back, while the patients observe themselves and their reactions to the trauma. The patients are then asked what new information was obtained from "watching the movie," especially information that related to their survival, and then asked to share that information with the "younger self," who had experienced the trauma. Theoretically, the separation, or disassociation, of the traumatic memory from its negative emotion occurs at this point and results in significant reduction of that emotion with future recall of the traumatic event.

The process involved in VKD must be differentiated from that of dissociation as discussed in Chapter 8. Dissociation entails a lack of integration into consciousness of a memory, emotion, or somatic experience. Disassociation in VKD involves an attempt to separate a traumatic memory from its associated negative emotion, and thereby isolate the memory from distress in the future.

TFT, an unusual technique devised by Callahan,[31] is based on a theory that "perturbations" in the "thought field"—i.e., any negative emotion, phobia, or anxiety—cause disruption in the body's energy system. This state of energy imbalance is measurable through a diagnostic process of strength testing based on the technique of applied kinesiology, which in turn is related to the concepts of meridian energy flow on which acupuncture is based. The treatment involves instructing the patient to tap strategic acupuncture meridian points determined by the diagnostic procedure, while simultaneously imaging or remembering a traumatic event, memory, phobia, or emotion. Frequently the process is blocked by "psychological reversals," a presumed reversal of a meridian polarity. These reversals are then corrected by tapping on the outside of the hand while saying three times, "I fully accept myself even though I have this problem." The patient then goes through a nine-step procedure involving a ritualized combination of eye movements, counting, and humming a few bars of a song while performing hand tapping. During this process, the patient's self-assessed SUDS rating is documented sequentially, with the goal being reduction of the scale to a 1.

The arcane nature of TFT, its radical departure from any standard concept of psychotherapy, and the supposed "quick fix" that it provides have predictably exposed it to the condemnation and ridicule of many research psychologists. These very features, however, have probably contributed to its remarkably widespread use by community-based psychotherapists frustrated by treatment failures with standard therapy for PTSD, and also to the success of Callahan's training seminars.

TIR is, in part, based on the assumption that traumatic memory contains gaps that may be important to the understanding and meaning of the memory, and may account for the distress associated with it. Frank Gerbode, the founder of TIR, believes that patients form an "intention" to resist the trauma, resulting in their inability to resolve it.[32] With the guidance of a therapist, the patient is instructed to visualize a traumatic event and to analyze it from beginning to end. The patient then reports the experience in detail to the therapist. The patient is guided by generally generic questions about the trauma, with no interpretative or evaluative statements being made by the therapist. The process is then repeated as many times as it takes to reach a "resolution," an event determined to have occurred by positive cues from the patient's behavior or verbalization, usually signaling relief, insight, or pleasant surprise.

The process is considered by Gerbode to be educational rather than therapeutic, a means of achieving personal growth rather than therapeutic healing. The treatment is open-ended, and may take ten to twenty repetitions to achieve resolution. Other traumatic events may then be followed in sequential sessions, reducing distress with each event until the core trauma is accessed. This gradual format theoretically protects against flooding. Unlike the other "power therapies," TIR seems to relate more to a relatively unstructured form of verbal psychotherapy, although its relatively simplistic and formulaic design suggests features of desensitization.

Anecdotal reports of dramatic "cures" through application of the power therapies are noted throughout published literature and meeting presentations, but as we have noted, scientific validation is lacking. Criticisms of these treatments include attribution of positive results to the power of suggestion, the placebo effect, and results analogous to faith healing. Nevertheless, all of these techniques incorporate the role of exposure to the traumatic memory in a relatively controlled environment, a technique currently thought to likely be the most effective mode of treatment of PTSD. This fact alone might explain some of the apparent effectiveness of the power therapies. In addition, the role of trust and of patient/therapist interaction is believed to constitute an important element in the success of psychotherapy.

Although there are many theories accounting for the efficacy of various psychotherapy techniques involving counseling and verbal interaction between therapist and patient, there really is no way to eliminate the effect of the placebo response in this relationship. In fact, the joint sharing of belief between therapist/physician and patient, that they are working together to achieve healing, is basically what constitutes the placebo response.[33] The power of suggestion in a therapeutic relationship can have powerful and measurable physical effects, both positive and negative.[34]

One must also consider that the clinical profile of the patient population likely to benefit from such techniques is highly weighted toward the dissociative and somatization disorders, both of which are common late expressions of PTSD. Patients with somatization disorders basically experience embodiment of emotions of distress through physical symptoms, are more likely to seek reassurance from the physician/therapist concerning the meaning of these symptoms ("effort after meaning"), and are more likely to benefit from their positive interaction—i.e., from the placebo effect. Dismissal of the efficacy of these techniques on this basis, therefore, is to criticize every psychotherapeutic technique ever devised.

Several other areas of major concern have been raised, especially with EMDR and TFT. These concerns relate to the peculiar nature of the concurrent physical stimuli provided with imaginal exposure, and with the basic concept of a rapid and dramatic therapeutic effect. Neither of these specific features of EMDR and TFT have any other historical precedents in methods of psychotherapy, except perhaps for the use of electroconvulsive therapy (ECT) for the treatment of major depression. They also do not relate to any treatment model for physical disease in the Western allopathic system of medicine. Rapid reversal of symptoms of disease through repetitive and somewhat ritualistic performance of prescribed motor activities by the therapist or the patient lends itself far more to folk or shamanic medicine than to anything to which allopathic therapists can relate. In other words, given our current paradigms, these exercises make no sense.

Cannon provides insight into the role that rituals play in human physiology in his exploration of the phenomenon of voodoo deaths in what we consider to be primitive cultures.[35] In voodoo death, an alteration of the basic physiology of a person who is subjected to a voodoo curse is caused by a series of rituals that tend to isolate the person from other members of the community, and which are associated in that culture with impending death. As the curse progresses, the patient lapses into torpor, and will eventually sink into a coma and die. The mode of death strongly suggests a state of profound parasympathetic tone, analogous to the freeze response, and perhaps mediated by profound tonic influence of the dorsal vagal complex (DVC, see Chapter 8). This state is induced entirely by the culturally determined meaning of the rituals to which the person is exposed. Conversely, a series of rituals, or counter charm, by the shaman or medicine man may actually reverse the entire process, and restore the person afflicted by the curse to health, again apparently through the *meaning* of the healing rituals.

I suspect that proponents of the power therapies would strongly object to the equation of their methods to shamanic ritualistic healing. The point that I would like to make, however, is that the performance of stylized rituals of healing in a primitive culture is based on generations of experience related to outcomes of treatment for specific symptoms and specific diseases, using very specific learned healing exercises. Not unlike EMDR and TFT, these ritualistic exercises are discovered and expanded through trial and error until a reasonable state of refinement is achieved. Since these treatments seem to be linked to a learned meaning of the procedure on a cultural basis, the brain and its effect on the stricken person almost certainly play a critical role in healing. If we continue to abide by the premise of the continuity of mind, brain, and body, then it is likely that this healing takes place through altered neurophysiology and neurochemistry. The very specific nature of such rituals also suggests that this brain/body effect cannot be achieved by any random nuance of behavior by the shaman, but only by those practices that have been found to alter the physiology of persons stricken with a curse.

Attempting to find the "active ingredients" in these unusual methods of treatment appears to be a worthwhile pursuit. However disparate they may appear to be, there may be a common neurophysiological thread that connects them in theory and effect. The burgeoning application of psychotropic and anticonvulsant drugs to the treatment of PTSD certainly supports the widely accepted concept that PTSD is a "physioneurosis."[36]

All mental illness must no longer be considered solely on the basis of the psychodynamics that led to the aberrant symptom complex. Rather, one must consider the neurophysiological basis for the dysfunctional behavior due to experienced-induced changes in neural structure. The unconscious and conditioned nature of much of PTSD symptomatology remains a powerful impetus to the development of treatment models that incorporate basically unconscious methods of extinction, desensitization, and quenching.

The search for treatment tools that may alter dysfunctional behavior by changing reflex patterns and neuronal pathways through unconscious methods of access to procedural memory and arousal systems has great appeal. These considerations clearly call for validation of somatically based techniques through appropriate studies, including attempts at dismantling the peculiar physical tools used in TFT, EMDR, and other similar reflexive therapies. Arbitrary dismissal of a technique as being too strange to be real, however, presumes that we know more about the brain, body, and behavior than we probably do.

PHARMACOTHERAPY OF POST-TRAUMATIC STRESS DISORDER

The compelling reemergence of Kardiner's concept of PTSD as a "physioneurosis"[36] might lead one to predict a flood of clinical studies examining the use of strategic pharmacological agents in the treatment of PTSD. Surprisingly, this has not been the case. Much of the research examining the use of medications for the arousal and avoidance symptoms of PTSD has been in the form of case studies and open-ended clinical drug trials. Randomized controlled trials (RCT) have been rare. Several factors have probably contributed to this problem. PTSD is a multifaceted biphasic disorder, characterized by a number of quite disparate criteria (arousal, avoidance/numbing, reexperiencing), and associated with a group of equally varied late clinical expressions (dissociation, affect dysregulation, depression, somatization). Many studies predictably document a relative specificity of the clinical efficacy of specific medications for the various manifestations of the syndrome. This conundrum of drug/symptom specificity, however, is quite consistent with the probability that different neurotransmitters may contribute to each of the many expressions of this disorder. Although a given patient may fulfill the DSM-IV criteria for PTSD, his or her clinical manifestations may be strongly biased in the direction of one particular symptom complex, such as arousal or numbing. As a result, in a given treatment trial, the clinical response may vary considerably from other verified PTSD patients with differing symptom dominance.

Any physician attempting to manage the varied symptoms of PTSD is well aware of the problem of precipitating anxiety and arousal through the use of a serotonin reuptake inhibitor (SRI), or compounding numbing or depression with an anxiolytic agent. The kindled sensitivity to any ambient sensory stimulus and the tendency to experience arousal or anxiety through somatic symptoms also renders these patients exquisitely sensitive to medication side effect, whether real or actually related to other ambient environmental stimuli. Under these conditions, not only the treatment but also the valid scientific study of drug efficacy in PTSD is extremely difficult. Despite these constraints, many open-ended drug trials have demonstrated strikingly beneficial clinical effects by a variety of medications for specific PTSD symptoms. As one would expect, application of early trial use of a medication has usually involved the administration of that drug for a symptom of PTSD that is similar to the symptom for which the drug is customarily prescribed. In general, the main medications studied and used in PTSD have fallen into the categories of anxiolytics, antidepressants and mood modulators.

Anxiolytic medications have included the benzodiazepines and buspirone. Brain receptors that bind the benzodiazepines are linked to the receptors for the inhibitory neurotransmitter, gamma amino butyric acid (GABA). One role of GABA, and therefore of the benzodiazepines, appears to be the control and modulation of anxiety.[37] Benzodiazepines might also play a role in modulating kindling, a compelling model for PTSD, since increase in benzodiazepine receptor binding is noted in experimental models of kindling.[38] Although this class of drugs has been used extensively in PTSD, few RCT clinical studies have been done to document their efficacy. In addition, there is general concern among clinicians about withdrawal symptoms from benzodiazapines associated with rebound anxiety, insomnia, aggression, and exacerbation of PTSD symptoms.[39,40] This is especially true for the short-acting benzodiazepines such as alprazolam. On the other hand, several open-ended studies have indicated efficacy of alprazolam and clonazepam in PTSD.[40,41] Much of this success, however, is thought to represent only reduction in anxiety-related symptoms. Clonazepam may represent an optimal agent in this drug class because of its lower habituation potential and its antikindling role as a primary anticonvulsant.

Buspirone is an anxiolytic agent with serotonergic properties, acting primarily as a 5-HT-1A partial agonist. It has a delayed onset of action, much like the SRI group of antidepressants. The limited research available concerning its efficacy suggests that it may improve symptoms of arousal, reexperiencing, and sleep impairment, but that it does not affect symptoms of avoidance or numbing.[42]

Tricyclic antidepressants (TCAs) have been subjected to the most utilization and clinical study in PTSD. Members of this class of drugs variably have both serotonergic and adrenergic actions, with suggestive evidence that those TCAs with the most serotonergic activity may be somewhat more effective. Because of the extremely frequent comorbidity of depression with PTSD, the fact that the major benefit of all of the antidepressant class of drugs may primarily be due to improvement in depression alone must always be considered.[43] RCTs with amitriptyline, a TCA with strong SRI effects, reveal moderate efficacy in improving symptoms of PTSD including depression and anxiety.[43,44]

Imipramine has also been shown to exhibit effectiveness in the treatment of PTSD in a number of RCTs, with its major area of benefit being reduction of symptoms of intrusion and reexperiencing, with less benefit observed in symptoms of avoidance.[45,46] Patients with major depression were excluded from the imipramine studies, lessening the likelihood that the therapeutic effects were primarily due to improvement in depression. Desipramine, a purely adrenergic TCA, was found to be little more effective than placebo in treatment of PTSD.[47]

The TCAs, of course, have a side-effect spectrum and incidence that is diverse and common enough to limit their use in these highly sensitive patients. In my experience, weight gain is extremely common in those patients with substantial symptoms of PTSD after motor vehicle accidents. The common association of this weight gain with an acneiform rash suggests that early hypersecretion of cortisol as part of the hormonal modulation and adaptation to trauma may trigger both of these problems. As a result, the additional weight gain common to the TCAs compounds this problem and further limits their long-term use in PTSD. Perhaps the most useful application of the TCAs to this disorder is their use in extremely low doses as a medication promoting sleep maintenance, an extremely common problem in PTSD. Although widely used in this capacity, their efficacy in sleep maintenance has not been specifically documented by the results of adequate RCTs.

Monoamine oxidase inhibitors (MAOIs) have been used and studied in PTSD to a limited extent but have not been widely applied due to the serious nature of their side effects. One well-designed RCT compared imipramine, phenelzine (an MAOI), and placebo.[46] Phenelzine was the most effective of the three treatments, with significant improvement noted in symptoms of intrusion and avoidance. In general, however, most clinicians reserve the use of MAOIs in PTSD to cases that have proven refractory to other safer medications.

Anticonvulsant medications have been applied to the treatment of PTSD with a similar rationale and in much the same fashion as they are applied to the treatment of bipolar disorder. The neurophysiological model of kindling has been applied on a theoretical basis to both conditions, and has generated increasing use of the newer anticonvulsant medications as mood modulators. The most commonly used anticonvulsants in PTSD are carbamazepine and valproate, both of which have been studied in open trials. Carbamazepine-treated veterans showed reduction in the severity of symptoms of arousal and intrusion, with improvement in flashback experiences and sleep quality.[48] Valproate-treated veterans also showed improvement in arousal and avoidant symptoms, but little in intrusion.[49] Other case studies generally showed comparable results but were marred by inclusion of patients with partial complex seizures, and by noting improvement in irritability and aggressive behavior without specifically addressing issues of PTSD symptoms. Newer anticonvulsant agents, including gabapentin and lamotrigine, have been used in PTSD with efficacy in anecdotal unpublished reports, but have not been subjected to formal study in open trials or RCTs. Gabapentin is unique in its remarkably benign side effect spectrum, its wide dose range and tolerance, and its freedom from apparent dependence or overdose risk. These features alone might raise skepticism about its actual effectiveness, but it appears to have achieved wide application in PTSD, chronic pain, and as a primary mood modulator. Its long-term efficacy as an antikindling agent in PTSD remains to be formally studied.

Alpha$_2$- and beta-adrenergic blocking agents have demonstrated some degree of efficacy in reducing symptoms of arousal in selected PTSD patients. One would expect a reduction in the perception of the physical symptoms of arousal based on blocking of the somatic end organs affected by adrenaline release with this class of drugs, and this effect might reduce the anxiety cascade associated with panic. The beta-blocker propranolol has been found to reduce a wide spectrum of arousal-based symptoms (hypervigilence, aggression, enhanced startle, intrusion, nightmares) in a varied population of PTSD victims, including combat veterans[50] and abused children.[51] Clonidine, an alpha$_2$-adrenergic antagonist, reduces adrenergic tone through a different mechanism than propranolol, but would be expected to have similar effects on arousal and anxiety. Like propranolol, clonidine has had some success in anxiety states. In a study with Vietnam veterans with PTSD, Kolb, Burris, and Griffiths,[50] documented therapeutic effects with clonidine similar to those noted with propranolol. Improvement in arousal symptoms of PTSD with administration of clonidine in children,[52] and in combination with imipramine in Cambodian refugees,[53] has also been noted in open trials. Side effects of both classes of drugs include bradycardia, hypotension, depression, and constipation, and are dose-limiting but usually manageable. Nevertheless, even open trial studies of this class of medicines have been rare despite promising results in the few published articles. Both classes of adrenergic blockers have clear application in PTSD patients who develop sustained elevation of blood pressure following trauma. Although sustained hypertension in these cases probably also stems from separate and additional risk factors, the use of adrenergic blockers as an approach to both problems has particular appeal.

Serotonin reuptake inhibitors (SRIs) have been studied and applied more extensively in PTSD than other agents, and appear to represent the most effective drugs for the treatment of this disorder. Although a number of open drug trials suggest that fluoxetine is effective in improving symptoms of intrusion, avoidance, and arousal, the most widely quoted RCT suggested that fluoxetine is uniquely effective in improving numbing, a symptom generally resistant to many of the other drugs studied.[54] This study by van der Kolk and colleagues also showed improvement in arousal, but less so in avoidant symptoms. In addition, fluoxetine improved associated symptoms of PTSD, including affect dysregulation, and the distortion of interpersonal relationships. Depression, however, was not significantly improved, suggesting that fluoxetine possesses a specific anti-PTSD effect. Recent FDA approval of sertraline as the first medication specifically indicated for the treatment of PTSD was based on two multicenter studies, both of which are still in press at the time of this writing. Findings were reviewed in the *PTSD Research Quarterly* by Friedman, and reflected previous findings that the SRIs tend to positively affect all three categories of PTSD symptoms (numbing, hyperarousal, reexperiencing).[55]

Narcotic antagonists have been applied to the treatment of PTSD in several studies based on the demonstration that arousal-induced analgesia was reversible by the narcotic antagonist, naloxone, when Vietnam veterans were exposed to combat scenes.[56] The emotional numbing of PTSD has been attributed to endorphin release associated with the traumatic experience.[57] This theory is consistent with theories of altered regulation of the endogenous opioid system in PTSD, and the role of opioid dysregulation in dissociation and the phenomenon of reenactment (see Chapters 7 and 8). However, an open study of the experimental opiate inhibitor nalmefene in Vietnam veterans produced improvement in numbing in less than half, and worsened anxiety and panic symptoms in a number of subjects.[58] A single case study also demonstrated reduction in traumatic flashbacks in two patients with the narcotic antagonist naltrexone.[59] These studies illustrate the dilemma in pharmacotherapy of PTSD related to the spectrum of symptoms at both extremes of arousal. Although fluoxetine also has been shown to diminish numbing in a number of patients, it may also precipitate anxiety and hyperarousal. One would expect the same to be true of narcotic antagonists, since numbing and dissociation are defensive reflex responses to the arousal generated by any threat in the PTSD patient.

CONCLUSION

This chapter has been an admittedly brief and basic overview of therapy for PTSD as it exists at the present time. The basic principles of treatment have been addressed in many chapters and review articles.[9,12,60] Although our expanding knowledge of the neurophysiological substrates of this diverse syndrome has provided a variety of logical constructs for treatment, the remarkable variation in symptoms both within individual patients, and among different patients with the disorder, seems to limit consistent successful therapeutic approaches to the problem. One is often left with such terms as "processing," "consolidating," "controlling," and "anxiety management" as means of handling an out-of-control autonomic flood. Social and personal attachments provide means of resource and support and are meant, along with these other generic concepts, to keep a finger in the dike of the always-threatened emotional deluge. Although researchers and clinicians who have devoted their lives to the study of PTSD recognize that emotional numbing remains the elusive white rabbit of trauma, the therapeutic key to dispelling dissociation and numbing remains an enigma. On the other hand, many victims of traumatic stress do respond to existing therapies, and many others rise above their panic and pain and reconstitute a reasonable semblance of emotional stability. Hopefully, the increasing awareness of the fact that the mind and the emotions in PTSD, and for that matter in all mental illness, reflect an ultimately identifiable and measurable aberration of brain physiology may lead to more specific, comprehensive, and rational treatment paradigms. Optimally, increasing recognition of the neglected role of somatically based symptoms in trauma will lead to integration of somatically based therapeutic techniques into the treatment mix.

Chapter 11

Case Histories:
The Somatic Spectrum of Trauma

I have already included a number of case studies in this book to illustrate several concepts of trauma in MVAs, especially related to the syndrome of somatic dissociation. I believe that a chapter devoted only to such stories will help to give a better picture of the wide range of symptoms of trauma, not only those categorized in the DSM-IV, but also those accompanying the late manifestations of trauma. The spectrum of unusual and varied symptoms in many of my patients paints a vivid and arresting portrait of trauma and the physical and emotional toll that it takes on the brains and bodies of its victims.

A STATE OF VULNERABILITY

My first case history is that of a young man, injured in a most unusual accident in a grocery store, which in other circumstances would have been considered trivial. A six-foot-four-inch, thirty-year-old man, he had the bulky upper body of a weight lifter. Yet when he spoke, his voice was soft and tentative. He took great pride in his body and health, pursuing fitness through exercise, and health through an organic, vegetarian diet. He told his story of trauma with obvious great distress. While shopping at a local health food store, he passed a display of stacked boxes of crackers, piled to a height of almost eight feet. At that moment, a box of crackers probably weighing five to eight pounds fell off of the top of the stack, hitting him on the back of his shoulders and neck. He was immediately stunned, and felt shocked and confused. Store personnel assisted him to a chair, where he remained for almost two hours, unable to pull himself out of a sense of shock and detachment. An on-site massage therapist gave him a massage, and the store provided an ice pack and juice to drink. He was finally able to pull himself together and called a friend for a ride home. Although he had no bruising or other signs of injury, over the next weeks he developed a syndrome of headaches, neck pain and muscle spasm, panic attacks, flashbacks and nightmares, depression, and impairment of memory.

When I saw him four months after the accident, his symptoms were becoming worse, and he had begun to have flashback memories of childhood trauma. He was the child of a physically abusive father; the parents had separated when he was five years old. At age six, his father broke into their home, shot him and his mother, and critically wounded both. He had only vague and disjointed memories of that traumatic event, but previously absent memories emerged in the face of his new, seemingly trivial traumatic experience in his thirties. Further evidence of his pervasive traumatic amnesia was found in the numerous scars on his body, the causes of which he had no memory.

This patient's case illustrates several principles in understanding traumatization. As in most cases of PTSD, distortions of memory in this patient were characterized by both traumatic amnesia and flashbacks. Flashbacks, nightmares, and intrusive thoughts represent exaggerated repetition of traumatic memory, and are part of the kindled cycle of arousal and memory seen in PTSD. Traumatic amnesia is dissociative in nature, and is typical of childhood trauma, in which dissociation is almost a universal response to trauma. Individuals traumatized in childhood continue to dissociate as adults when exposed to trauma, even when the trauma is relatively trivial, as in this case.

As perhaps the most potent predictor for the development of PTSD, dissociation in this case of unusual trauma led to full-blown PTSD that persisted for months, and was severe enough to resurrect old traumatic memories and PTSD related to childhood trauma. The patient's attempts to build personal resources through his compulsively health-oriented lifestyle were no match for the unstable autonomic and neurophysiological mechanisms for dealing with any new stress resulting from his horrible childhood experiences. In addition, the traumatic event that triggered PTSD in his case certainly did not constitute a criterion for traumatization as defined in the DSM-IV.

Low-velocity MVAs also do not fulfill this criterion, but may result in severe traumatization in selected cases. Clearly the *meaning* of the precipitating event must be considered when determining whether a person has been traumatized. In cases in which the victim has a past history of multiple or severe traumatic life events, especially in childhood, a seemingly trivial threat may be perceived as life threatening. Individuals with childhood trauma seem to lack the resiliency to deal with later traumatic stress, and easily decompensate under relatively minor stressful events. When confronted with a patient with a disproportionate emotional response to a stressful event, a careful history of life trauma will usually reveal events that clearly explain the remarkable vulnerability exhibited by them.

SOMATIC REPRESENTATIONS OF PRIOR TRAUMA

A second case study also illustrates the role of past life trauma in establishing a meaning for subsequent life events, which, although superficially trivial, may prove to be profoundly traumatizing. A female patient of mine in her twenties presented with a history of having visited a new chiropractor for an adjustment. The chiropractor took the patient's head between his hands and performed significant quick rotational adjustment more violent than she was used to. The patient immediately experienced a sense of shock and horror and told the therapist, who apologized and continued with a more gentle manipulation. That night the patient experienced increasing headache, nausea, and cervical muscle spasm. She returned the next day to the chiropractor, hoping for some relief from her pain. After examining her, the chiropractor indicated that he could "fix" her neck, and once again performed a ballistic adjustment. At this point, the patient experienced uncontrolled panic and left the office acutely agitated and in great pain.

Over the next two weeks, she developed severe headaches, cervical spasm, blurred vision, photophobia, nausea, vertigo, confusion, and memory loss. She was hypervigilant with exaggerated startle, and experienced flashbacks of the therapy and of old childhood trauma. She experienced severe nightmares and sleep disturbance. Cognitive symptoms in the form of forgetfulness, distraction, and episodes of confusion soon appeared. At the time of her first visit to my office, the

patient wore a cervical collar. She was able to move her head by herself to a limited degree, but when I attempted to test that motion by
moving her head gently with my hands, her neck was completely
rigid. Neck movement caused nausea and vertigo. Nonphysiological
give-away weakness, glove-distribution sensory loss, and dramatic
pain behavior were prominent. Her syndrome could well have been
consistent with a whiplash experience in a patient prone to somatization. Her psychosocial history, however, revealed that as a child
of eight she had been subjected to repeated incest by a male relative
who achieved compliance by partial strangulation with his arm around
her neck as a means of control.

In many cases of seemingly trivial injuries leading to PTSD, the
key to the puzzle is found in the somatic representations of both prior
trauma and/or the precipitating traumatic event. The somatic association with the neck in this case is obvious. Once again, traumatic
events incorporating the head or neck seem particularly potent with
regard to trauma potential (see Chapter 4). This case also illustrates
that the whiplash syndrome consists of a reproducible constellation
of symptoms that may have nothing to do with an MVA. This syndrome includes not only regional myofascial pain, but also cognitive
impairment typical of minor brain injury in the absence of any possible brain injury. A threat to one's life and resulting helplessness certainly occurred in this case, but only if one took into account the
meaning of the presumed traumatic event in the form of the region of
the body involved in the experience.

Another simple example of the retention of procedural memory for
prior trauma-induced pain concerned a middle-aged woman involved in
a moderate velocity rear-end MVA. Months later, she presented to
me with persistent pain underneath her left scapula. Examination revealed typical findings of taut, tender muscles in the area of her persistent pain. Upon palpating these painful muscles, she suddenly
cried out in great distress. I apologized for apparently having been too
vigorous in my examination. She, however, said that it was not my
fault, but that she suddenly had a flash of insight that the area of pain
was the spot that "the nuns used to hit me." As a child in a Catholic
boarding school, the nuns supervising the students made it a habit to
discipline their charges by confronting them unannounced while the
students were in their evening bath, striking them with a switch for
perceived misdeeds that day. Because of the position of the tub, my

patient invariably received her punishing blows under the left scapula. Procedural memory for this frightening and dreaded experience remained stored for future reference in her survival brain, and was reactivated by the experience of a new life threat, her MVA.

MEDICAL AND FORENSIC RETRAUMATIZATION

Unfortunately, physical injuries resulting in traumatization often are associated with incorporation of the legal system in attempts to resolve issues of causation and validity. Such is the case in MVAs, athletic injuries, falls, and various types of assault, including rapes and muggings. Because patients with prior life trauma are disproportionately vulnerable to retraumatization, their overt emotional and somatic response to injury may appear inappropriately severe. These patients are often soon labeled by the medical profession as being "overresponders," suffering from psychophysiological problems, or exhibiting secondary gain behavior. Personnel handling their case for their auto or health insurance company soon access this information and begin to question the validity of the injury. Feeling invalidated by their own physician and health care insurance provider, the traumatized patients soon seek legal advice. The cycle of mistrust, skepticism, invalidation, fear, and frustration thereafter serves to perpetuate the patient's symptoms as a self-fulfilling prophecy.

Many of my patients have experienced this dilemma to some extent. One in particular exemplifies this problem, as well as a number of other unusual features of trauma. A female accountant, she was driving a client home when an argument ensued. The client had a history of bipolar mental illness, became agitated and paranoid, and began to strike the woman on the right shoulder and head. Swerving to the left, the woman saw an oncoming truck, swerved to the right, and ran off the road into a ditch. The accident was at low velocity and did not damage the car or, apparently, its occupants. The assaultive client at that point left the car, and walked across the field to his home.

Although she appeared uninjured, the patient rapidly developed severe right neck, shoulder, and arm pain and underwent several years of therapy with limited improvement. She experienced the onset of severe cognitive symptoms after a delay of about six weeks, was diagnosed with a closed head injury, and received prolonged cognitive therapy. Anxiety and panic, flashbacks, intrusive thoughts of the attack and accident, and nightmares developed. She received psychotherapy and was given trials of many psychotropic medications. When I saw her, a trauma history revealed that throughout childhood her father had been physically abusive to the family to the extent that at age twenty-one, the patient was actually hospitalized after a beating. She had not seen or spoken to him since then.

Despite ongoing pain, weakness, and numbness of the right arm, as well as cognitive and emotional impairment, the patient had resumed working. I referred her for somatically based trauma therapy after interpreting her symptoms for her, and she had a remarkable resolution of virtually all of these symptoms. Especially notable was the clearing of most attention and memory deficits. Symptoms of pain and PTSD largely subsided.

As her legal case progressed, however, she was subjected to a series of independent medical examinations (IMEs), including repeated neuropsychological test batteries. Faced once again with skepticism and challenges to the validity of her injury, some of her symptoms of arousal began to reemerge. After a confrontational and adversarial deposition by opposing lawyers, she returned to see me with a full-blown recurrence of all of her cognitive, emotional, and somatic symptoms. A repeat course of therapy and settlement of her case out of court for a trivial amount resulted in improvement of symptoms once again, and she has subsequently done well. Her recovery was clearly related to the cessation of hostilities with the legal and insurance industries, and not to secondary gain.

Had this patient been recognized from the start as a victim of trauma, with a valid and predictable syndrome based on the nature of the accident, and had appropriate trauma therapy been instituted early, medical cost savings would likely have been achieved. More important, however, the serial and repetitive retraumatization by medical, insurance, and legal systems would likely not have occurred, and her state of vulnerability to subsequent trauma would not have been enhanced. A careful history would have determined that the attack by her passenger, and not the MVA itself, was the source of trauma, based on her childhood physical abuse.

This patient represents dozens of my patients whose syndromes of trauma have been perpetuated or resurrected in this manner. My interactions with insurance adjustors and nurse case managers have revealed a deep-seated mistrust of patients who carry the diagnosis of "soft tissue injuries," "minor traumatic brain injury," or "whiplash." Understandably, this is based on the dilemmas posed in Chapters 3 and 4. Many physicians share this disdain for the validity of these symptoms and diagnoses. Some have chosen to take advantage of this bias and voluntarily seek the role of performing IMEs for automobile and liability insurance companies, often at great profit. Predictably many such IME reports are demeaning and critical of the validity of the patient's complaints, and contribute to perpetuating sequential retraumatization of the patient. Because our system of jurisprudence is by definition adversarial, the prescribed sequence of legal events in an MVA insurance claim predictably enhances symptoms of trauma, prolongs the patient's illness, and jeopardizes the outcome. In virtually every case of delayed whiplash recovery due to traumatization, I eventually spend more time treating the patient for effects of stress from the insurance and legal systems than for the original accident.

MULTIPLE CHEMICAL SENSITIVITIES

Another example of the appearance of cognitive and emotional symptoms in the absence of velocity-related injury occurred in a patient of mine who presented as a case of chronic carbon monoxide poisoning. Three months after moving into a new house, the patient, a middle-aged woman, developed a syndrome of intractable nausea, cramps, and urinary and fecal incontinence with subsequent negative medical evaluations. She then developed distal tingling of her hands, blurring of vision, impaired memory and attention, apathy, panic attacks, and depression. Diffuse muscular pain ensued, and one year after the onset of symptoms, elevated carbon monoxide levels were found in her house due to a defective furnace.

Despite correction of the defect, her emotional and cognitive symptoms worsened and she developed a peculiar slurred and stuttering speech pattern several months after the exposure. MRI of the brain and EEG were normal, as was her neurological examination except for a clearly nonphysiological stutter. All symptoms and signs fluctuated dramatically, in direct proportion to incidental life stress.

The entire symptom complex nevertheless progressed to the point of complete disability, and she applied for Social Security disability.

Her past medical history included a long record of recurrent myofascial low back and neck pain, carpal tunnel, and thoracic outlet syndromes, the latter two conditions leading to surgery. She had been treated in a clinic for chronic pain. At age eight, she had experienced a prolonged hospitalization for pelvic and femoral fractures, and at age five, she suffered multiple episodes of sexual molestation by a babysitter. Her one marriage was associated with spousal abuse and ended in divorce.

This patient clearly demonstrates the typical pattern of symptoms of late effects of trauma, many of which are typical of delayed recovery in whiplash. Although it might be tempting to relate her neurological syndrome to brain injury from low-level exposure to carbon monoxide, injuries of this sort are unproven. In addition, delayed appearance of neurological symptoms following acute exposure to toxic levels of carbon monoxide is usually severe and often fatal, usually involving brain white matter lesions on the MRI.

On the other hand, diffuse somatic, emotional, and cognitive symptoms, including those of PTSD, have been described in the syndrome of multiple chemical sensitivities (MCS).[1,2] Several investigators have postulated the role of neurosensitization or kindling in the etiology of MCS.[1,2] These theories relate the close association between olfactory and limbic pathways in precipitating neurosensitization in such patients. Sensitivity to olfactory stimulation in the kindled trauma patient may well be related to the fact that olfaction is the only primary sense that accesses the limbic system without the filter of the thalamus. The patient described here may represent a case of unique vulnerability to autonomic arousal triggered by what might be considered a trivial exposure to olfactory stimuli. Multiple episodes of prior life traumatic stress had already caused many of the symptoms of late effects of traumatization, and led to an ongoing state of chronic neurosensitization, or kindling. Such a state typically is associated with increased sensitivity to arousal with even remotely negative environmental stimuli. Certainly the olfactory/limbic connection could lead to enhancement of kindling in such patients. An epidemiological study of the association of past life trauma with MCS certainly appears warranted.

THE MYSTERIOUS PIRIFORMIS

Piriformis syndrome (PS) has been described and discussed for seventy years. It has been defined as buttock and back pain with a positive Lesegue (straight leg raising) sign, tenderness at the sciatic notch, absence of neurological signs, and improvement with conservative therapy.[3] The piriformis muscle arises from the ventrolateral surface of the sacrum and sacroiliac joint, passes out of the sciatic notch, and inserts on the greater trochanter of the femur. It forms part of the posterior boundary of the pelvis, and is intimately associated with the branches of the sciatic nerve. As a result, true sciatica, or neurogenic pain running down the posterior thigh and calf, is frequently associated with the piriformis syndrome. The syndrome often follows a minor low back strain or overuse injury of the back, but also often occurs without apparent injury. It is associated with myofascial tightness, spasm, and shortening of the piriformis muscle. Incidence is considerably higher in women, with a ratio of 6:1 compared to men.[3] In women, pelvic pain and dyspareunia (painful intercourse) often accompany piriformis syndrome. Treatment includes standard physical therapy measures, including modalities such as heat, ice, and ultrasound, as well as specific stretching exercises. Local injections with steroids and/or local anesthetics may be useful, but are difficult due to the muscle's relatively deep location. In women, however, close association of the piriformis with the posterior vaginal wall allows easy transvaginal injection.

In my clinical experience with piriformis syndrome, I have typically noted the significant female preponderance of cases, most occurring in the context of falls, MVAs, or nonspecific back injuries. One such case started me on the investigation of prior life trauma in the role of piriformis syndrome, with startling results.

A young woman suffering neck and low back injuries from an MVA came to see me with prolonged and recalcitrant left sciatica. Although she was married, another female invariably accompanied her when she came to see me. (In my long clinical experience, when an adult woman always brings another woman with her to see me, a male doctor, there is a fairly high likelihood that she has experienced sexual trauma in her past.) The results of her examination, involving straight leg raising and strength testing, were consistent with the classic signs of piriformis syndrome, but remarkably the examination also caused her to become severely nauseated. She reported that this nausea often lasted for hours after she left my office, prompting me to discontinue my examinations at the time of her visits. Her past history was vague, but suggestive of some childhood trauma that I suspected was sexual in nature. The usual and appropriate physical therapy measures only made her worse, and she eventually did not return to see me.

Within the following year, I became interested in the role of trauma in the whiplash syndrome and myofascial pain, and developed some of the theories on which this book is based. As I began to take trauma histories in all of my patients with myofascial pain, I discovered a shocking association in my next thirty female patients and one male patient who presented with clinically consistent piriformis syndrome. All of these patients without exception had suffered sexual trauma, including childhood incest, rape, or molestation with penetration, or rape as an adult.

A paper studying these cases is pending publication, but several conclusions can be made from this association of a myofascial pain syndrome involving the piriformis syndrome in women and forced sexual penetration. The anatomical and kinesiological function of the piriformis muscle is external rotation of the femur. It also results in clenching of the buttocks and compression of the posterior pelvic wall. Its contraction is involved in the Kegel maneuver, an exercise used for strengthening the vaginal wall after childbirth and for shutting off the stream of urine. In the case of forced vaginal penetration, the piriformis clearly will be involved in the unconscious and reflexive protective neuromuscular response to the traumatic event. Unconscious piriformis contraction will, thereafter, be incorporated in the kindled circuitry of arousal, memory, and muscular bracing described in Chapter 4. Reminiscent life events, nonspecific stress or arousal, or repetitive use of the piriformis in a variety of situations may precipitate procedural memory for the defensive role of that muscle in past sexual trauma, and lead to its persistent contraction and spasm. In many cases, but obviously not all, I believe that the piriformis syndrome in women is an unusual and dramatic example of the traumatic basis for regional myofascial pain in a kindled neuromuscular reflex.

DISORDERS OF SPEECH IN TRAUMA

A number of my patients who have shown other signs of trauma after an MVA or other traumatic event have developed an unusual syndrome of delayed development of stereotyped disorders of articulation. The previously described patient with chronic carbon monoxide exposure manifested this symptom several months after she actually detected the smell of gas in her home. In virtually all of my other cases, the dysarthric speech disturbance also developed as a delayed event weeks or even months after the trauma. Onset of the speech disturbance was preceded by cognitive symptoms suggestive of a brain injury, as well as by criteria-based symptoms consistent with the diagnosis of post-traumatic stress disorder (PTSD). Most patients had a history of substantial prior life trauma.

One such patient, a middle-aged woman, was injured in a broadside MVA in which her husband was apparently unaffected. She may have experienced a brief period of unconsciousness, and was described by her husband as being confused on the way to the hospital. For several days she experienced only headache and stiff neck, but after several weeks, she developed increasing symptoms of dramatic stuttering, word blocking, and problems with attention and memory. Anxiety, photophobia, and sleep disturbance also appeared. She gradually developed right hand tremor, a right facial twitch, and squinting of her right eye. Her past history revealed a prior auto accident six years before characterized by prolonged spinal myofascial pain, with a prominent piriformis syndrome. She also had a history of cyclical depression.

Her initial physical examination by me six weeks after the accident revealed a dramatic stutter primarily with words starting with consonants. My impression was that the findings of my examination did not appear consistent with an organic pathological lesion of the brain. Indeed, MRI of the brain was normal.

The patient underwent a prolonged course of treatment, including cognitive therapy, physical therapy, and somatically based trauma therapy. Due to her stimulus sensitivity, she essentially remained confined to her house except for medical appointments. She experienced gradual improvement, with disappearance of the stutter, tremor, cognitive and emotional symptoms, and eventually was able to drive alone on side roads. Her agoraphobia related to being in public places when other people were present, however, remained disabling. Under such circumstances, all of her nonphysiological neurological symptoms, including her stutter, hand tremor, and facial twitch recurred.

Clinical features of speech abnormalities in the other patients have been remarkably similar to those described above. Most speech impediments have appeared, disappeared, or fluctuated in direct proportion to incidental life stress and to fatigue. The disorder is most often described as a stutter, or blockage of speech, and is associated with independent word blocking as well. A scanning, slurred, and dysarthric pattern is common, with independent prolongation of vowels, consonants, and diphthongs without any consistency. In one case, the patient developed what could be described only as a foreign or regional accent, with a consistent and reproducible pattern of mispronunciation. Onset of the speech impairment is usually delayed and recovery incomplete. Imaging studies of the brain have been routinely negative. Neuropsychological test batteries all show significant cognitive impairment consistent with minor traumatic brain injury (MTBI), PTSD, or both. In most cases, the speech abnormalities have been extremely resistant to treatment, and have persisted for years, usually in association with residual late symptoms of trauma.

The impairment in speech in these patients is clearly dissociative in nature, and might well be classified under the conversion disorders. In many instances, forces involved in the MVAs were relatively minor and inconsistent with production of an MTBI. Evaluation by speech pathologists routinely led to the conclusion that the speech disturbances were nonphysiological, and not consistent with any clear pathological process. All of the patients were women, and most of them had a history of prior trauma before the precipitating event. Although many carried the clinical diagnosis of MTBI, and all had cognitive dysfunction, symptoms of PTSD were uniformly prominent. The cyclical periods of improvement in speech invariably correlated with reduction of life stress and improvement in symptoms of trauma.

In the case history described, the patient had a past history of piriformis syndrome following another auto accident. A history of childhood trauma could not be obtained, although her neurological symptoms were clearly dissociative in nature. Perhaps the most salient clinical feature in these patients is the similarity of the quality of the speech impediment among patients. This rare but consistent association with traumatization suggests a common connection between areas of the brain linked to production of speech and the phenomenon of kindling involving areas of the brain linked to PTSD. The frequent concomitant occurrence of a tremor of the right hand or right facial twitch in these patients obviously has raised concerns about a structural left hemispheric lesion, but imaging studies have invariably been negative.

A group of patients with PTSD were read stories of their traumatic experience while positron-emission tomography (PET) scans of their brains were done. Heightened brain activity was noted in the right hemisphere, an area predictably linked to arousal and memory mechanisms associated with their trauma.[4,5] Broca's area for speech in the left hemisphere, however, showed abnormally diminished activity in these patients. Van der Kolk, and Rauch and colleagues postulate that this finding may explain alexithymia in traumatized patients: the inability to put feelings into words, and the tendency to experience emotions as physical states. In our cases of rare but stereotyped dysarthria in patients with PTSD, this phenomenon might also reflect changes in brain activity specific to the areas of the brain serving expressive speech that are inhibited by kindling and arousal activity in the right hemisphere. As we have noted, many patients with PTSD manifest simple word-finding difficulties. The dysarthric speech patterns observed in the patients described here may represent a further expression of the negative relationship between traumatic arousal and physiological suppression of metabolic function and circulatory patterns in Broca's area and related left hemispheric regions.

SPASMODIC TORTICOLLIS:
AN ABERRATION OF THE ORIENTING REFLEX

A woman came to see me for a second opinion regarding her long-standing involuntary head movements. At age three, she broke her left clavicle, and at fourteen, she suffered a broken nose and strained neck in a pool diving accident. During junior high school, she recalls having an occasional head twitch to the right without any change or worsening over the years. Then at age twenty-seven, she was involved in a catastrophic auto accident in which her husband was killed. For several hours, she was pinned in the car with her dead husband's head pinned against the left side of her head, forcing her head to the right.

Within months, she developed a persistent repetitive involuntary turning of her head to the right, diagnosed eventually by a neurologist as spasmodic torticollis. This head twitch was worsened by stress and emotion, and reduced by lightly touching the right side of her chin. Patching her left eye also partially corrected the head turning, a fact that she attributed to forcing her head to turn so that she could see straight ahead. The torticollis had not responded to a number of medications, and she was considering surgery, or possibly a trial of botulinum toxin injections. Her examination revealed spasmodic torsional movements of the head to the right, and the right ear to the right shoulder, quite typical of torticollis.

Because of the striking history of presumed traumatic origin of this patient's movement disorder, a course of somatic trauma therapy was instituted. After a fairly prolonged trial of therapy, the patient noted marked but incomplete improvement in the severity of her torticollis, with much of this improvement being due to the reduced effect of life stress on its severity. Pain due to the involuntary movement was substantially reduced.

Spasmodic torticollis is a focal dystonic movement disorder involving the head and neck of unknown cause, recognized for over a century, and generally resistant to treatment of any sort. In many cases, the cause has been felt to be due to psychogenic[6] or traumatic[7] factors, but psychotherapy and behavioral therapies have had mixed to poor results. Pain is common in up to 50 percent of cases and generally is associated with a poor prognosis.[7] Remission or improvement is common, but complete recovery is rare.[8] No pathology within the central nervous system has been demonstrated, and no specific cause has been found for torticollis.

The orientation response is a basic primitive sensorimotor reflexive response to perceived threat common to all animal species. Mobilization of the primary senses of smell, sight, and hearing for acquisition of potentially threatening sensory information involves orientation of those sensory end organs to the source of that information. This process involves neuromuscular control of the head and neck in order to position these organs for optimal sensory input. An animal perceiving a potential source of threat will exhibit immediate arrest of all movement, followed by a slow side-to-side scanning movement of the head associated with flaring of the nostrils, widening of the palpebral fissures, dilatation of the pupils, and forward rotation of the ears. These smooth turning movements of the head and neck in the direction of the threat orient the animal to the source of the arousal, and prepare it for defensive action. This reflexive sequence of movement is common to all species, and is triggered by the neurohumoral process of arousal. The orienting response very likely is mediated by the influence of the brainstem ventral vagal complex (VVC) as part of the energy-conserving, early behavioral response to arousal.[9]

Careful observation of patients who have experienced trauma will often reveal altered and sustained positions of the head and neck that reflect muscle-holding patterns representative of procedural memory for that trauma. Thus, the patient who has suffered injuries in a broadside, or T-bone automobile impact will usually present with a subtle, but quite obvious lateral shift and rotation of the head and neck in the direction away from the impact months and even years later. One may recall the patient described in Chapter 8 who had suffered severe injuries to the left arm, and whose posture was characterized by turning of the entire body away from the left side. These postures reflect orienting and defensive patterns of motor activity triggered by the threatening sensory input at the moment of a traumatic event, stored in procedural motor memory and linked to the arousal elicited by that event. Portions of these postures consist of the early orienting reflex involving scanning movements of the head as the initial response to possible threat. In the course of somatically based trauma therapy (such as Eye Movement Desensitization and Reprocessing, and Somatic Experiencing), subtle, to at times dramatic, involuntary turning movements of the head are elicited, presumably representing elicitation of orienting movements from procedural memory.

In the case of torticollis described previously, a series of traumatic experiences occurred in this patient that were specifically related to directional positioning of the head. The turning movements of the head in torticollis mimic in many respects those involved in the orientation response. Spasmodic torticollis, in fact, may be analogous to the bracing patterns of myofascial pain as a reflex movement pattern associated with a traumatic event locked in procedural memory in association with the arousal elicited by that event. As such, it may reflect a stereotyped repetitive orienting response perpetuated by traumatic kindling.

DISSOCIATION AND REFLEX
SYMPATHETIC DYSTROPHY

We have already discussed the syndrome of RSD in Chapters 6 and 8 in relationship to the concept of somatic dissociation, boundary rupture, and the role of the autonomic nervous system in its pathology. Recently, however, a patient presented to me with an uncanny validation of these concepts of the etiology of PTSD. The patient herself had an intuition that her doctor's explanations did not make sense in relationship to her personal experience, and she had formed her own theory of how this process had taken place. As a psychotherapist with a holistic view of the mind/body relationship, she decided that the traumatic experience itself and the meaning of events surrounding it must be related to her disease process.

While driving at moderate speed, her car was hit head-on by another automobile, and although her seat belt restraints prevented more severe injury, she suffered a major fracture injury to her right foot. She anticipated the impact before it occurred, and experienced severe auto-related PTSD that required years of psychotherapy to partially resolve.

While in the hospital awaiting surgery on her foot, she experienced intolerable pain despite narcotic administration. Using her acquired skills in the area of self-modulation and pain management, she utilized imaginary distancing of herself from the painful foot, visualizing that it indeed was not part of her. This was quite successful in reducing the intolerable portion of the pain, and she went on to have uneventful surgical repair of the foot fractures. Postoperative pain was severe, however, and once again became resistant to narcotic analgesia. When the cast was removed, the foot was gray and cold, and soon progressed to full-blown RSD.

In the next few years she underwent extensive pharmacotherapy, and over twenty-five sympathetic nerve blocks with only slight improvement in intractable burning foot pain. At some point in her recovery, she came to the conclusion that the act of her disowning the foot before surgery might indeed be related to her RSD. She then began an intensive program of imaging the blood vessels and temperature in her leg and foot, visualizing widening of the vessels, increase in blood flow and warmth. Although progress was slow, this practice began a gradual reversal of the dystrophy, pain, and hyperpathia of the RSD, and without further medical intervention, she largely recovered a normal foot except for mild hyperpathia and cold intolerance. Of interest is the fact that her pain syndrome also involved numbness and pain in the right jaw, face, arm, and hand, which gradually recovered.

Her physical examination at the time of her visit with me revealed no objective findings except for some residual tightness of muscles of the right shoulder girdle. With boundary testing, however, she experienced arousal and sudden pain in her right jaw when I passed my hand into her far right visual field at a distance of about four feet. This effect was quite startling to her, and reproducible on several trials. When I described to her my theory of RSD and how it exactly mimicked her process of intentional dissociation of her foot in the face of developing traumatization, she said that this actually was what she thought might have happened. She was afraid to tell her doctor, however, because the idea sounded so strange.

Since I have begun testing my patients for arousal symptoms within regions of their boundary perception, I have consistently found boundary rupture in RSD patients in the symptomatic region. Many of my RSD patients describe symptoms that might be interpreted as dissociation related to the initiating traumatic event. Many others develop RSD insidiously in the face of subtle injuries such as overuse of the hand, bumping part of the body, or suffering a minor sprain injury.

The aforementioned patient is obviously unique, not only in her powers of observation and self-control, but also in the 1:1 association of voluntary dissociation of the injured regions with subsequent development of RSD in the dissociated body part. A smoking gun at the scene of a crime is legal though not scientific proof, but it remains powerful evidence for an association.

COMMENTS

These stories illustrate a spectrum of somatic responses to traumatic stress that hopefully reinforce the basic premise of this book: the presence of a direct link between the neurochemical and neurophysiological response of the brain to stress, and an explainable, and measurable related somatic event. Using the symptoms and messages provided by apparent somatization as clues to the meaning of the patient's trauma, may allow the clinician to trace that message back to its source and thereby achieve greater understanding of the roots of the patient's illness. Although it would be presumptuous to assert that the truth will actually free the trauma victims from their autonomic bondage, self-knowledge through education and insight provided by the therapist remain powerful tools for providing resources for the patients throughout treatment. Understanding the links between their conditioned somatic and emotional response to internal and external sources of arousal may allow the patients to use self-regulatory skills attained through treatment to better advantage.

Establishing a relationship with a therapist that includes validation of the patient's physical symptoms as meaningful, measurable, and not "in one's head" lessens the ongoing stress of disbelief and devaluation by family, friends, health care providers, insurance personnel, and attorneys. Analysis of trauma-related postural changes, neurological symptoms, and boundary ruptures in relationship to the patient's trauma history may give valuable clues to which life trauma is the major perpetuating source of the patient's disability, and may provide valuable direction for the patient's treatment. Recognizing the true pathophysiological basis for the patient's symptoms may also facilitate treatment of the physical illnesses that may accompany and be attributable to traumatic stress.

Anecdotes such as these case histories do not make scientific fact. The role of coincidence and chance in the affairs of man and the universe have justifiably led to the role of the scientific method in determining truth in science. Unfortunately, medical science is among the least precise of sciences, and behavioral sciences are perhaps the least testable of all sciences. The brief review of the history of PTSD in psychiatry would certainly confirm this. Freud based his theories on his experience with thousands of patients, seasoned by a formidable intellect. He was not able to apply blinded controls to justify his conclusions. Nevertheless, before his views were warped by the need to succumb to the political pressures of his peers, he and Janet through patient observation alone had independently arrived at conclusions very close to our current psychophysiological theories of PTSD.

Similar to the anecdote of the four blind men and the elephant, we only believe in that part of the whole which we perceive, and what we perceive may be determined as much by secondary gain related to our role in the scientific community as by our search for the truth. The truth is actually out there in the brains and bodies of our patients. In our rush to science, we at times have substituted technology for science. We tend to trust that what we see in numbers, images, and measurements constitutes reality and, therefore, the truth. We have in part abandoned and allowed the use of our own senses and perceptions as healers to atrophy, the attributes that in the remote days of my training were valued as the essence of the true physician.

The greatest of these attributes is the spoken word expressed by the patient to his or her physician, where we often find the truth that we so desperately seek. That truth lies not only in the simplistic description of a physical symptom of an obvious disease, but also in the convoluted, tangential complaints associated with somatization. Dismissing a symptom or physical complaint because it "doesn't make sense" or is "psychological," imprisons the patient in a web of misunderstanding, and the physician in the bonds of bias. Our patients who suffer from the physiological ravages of trauma exemplify this fact more than any other patient group. They constitute the least understood, most rejected, and most frustrating challenges to the medical profession only because they represent a threat to our jaded concepts of tangible physical disease and intangible psychology. Once we reject this dichotomy, we will begin to recognize the remarkable physiological basis for "functional," "hysterical," "nonphysiological," and "psychosomatic" symptoms and physical findings, and we may recognize them as a part of a definable and reproducible syndrome, and approach treatment with understanding, empathy, and a healing spirit.

Postscript

We have arrived at a model of traumatization that I suspect will be intriguing and even compelling to some and, frankly, speculative to others. As our knowledge of the neurophysiological basis for PTSD expands, some elements of this theoretical model will undoubtedly change, and others I think will be validated. We have reemphasized the crucial role of dissociation in the perpetuation of the kindled autonomic cycle of PTSD. We have moved beyond the concept that somatic sensations have become a source of arousal in the PTSD victim, to the concept that these sensations represent actual physiological changes in the body region encompassing messages of the threat.

In this context, reexperiencing and dissociation driven by internal arousal cues have thrust the victim into a perceptual state locked in the past, incapable of experiencing the present, and blind to the future. Without the ability of the down-regulated frontal cortex to imagine "What if?" the future holds no other possibilities than existential threat. There can be no future while the unresolved procedural memories of the trauma continue to imply their ongoing and threatening presence. The ongoing cues of the present continue to trigger indiscriminate arousal and fear. The present, therefore, serves only to thrust the victim back into instinctual and conditioned modes of self-preservation that by definition are based on past failed attempts at escape and completion of the survival effort, and that only serve to enhance their sense of helplessness. Perhaps the most poignant complaint of the trauma victim is the loss of the sense of "who I was," and "who I am now." One's sense of self is not only based on the internal historical narrative of one's life experiences and accomplishments, but also on the ability to apply these experiences to future efforts. The perception of helplessness by definition belies this capability.

The therapeutic implications of these concepts are that healing in trauma will not be achieved until empowerment occurs, and until the ongoing threats and cues to arousal have been removed from a state of ongoing imminence to a state of past and completed experience.

Whether or not this experience encompasses a meaningful narrative may not be important, as long as the somatic correlates of the traumatic memory no longer contain messages of threat. Under this paradigm, the resolution of these somatic correlates may be the most important measure of successful trauma therapy.

* * *

During the preparation of this book, dramatic progress has been made in the study of the brain in PTSD. Among the most exciting areas of progress has been the use of imaging techniques in trauma victims to study brain metabolism and physiology in trauma victims. These studies have continued to demonstrate the selective facilitation and inhibition of areas of the brain known to participate in the cycle of traumatic kindling.

More attention has been directed at the role of childhood developmental experiences in the generation of personality, psychopathology, and vulnerability to trauma. Workers in the field of child development have begun to explore links between increasing childhood violence and more subtle issues of neglect and abandonment, such as the common use in the past decade of day care centers for children below the age of eighteen months. The association between such issues of early childhood experience and the development of attention deficit hyperactivity disorder (ADHD) is beginning to be addressed.

In the area of trauma therapy, more attention has been directed at somatically based trauma therapies, leading to a burgeoning growth of eclectic therapeutic approaches, many of them offshoots of existing therapies, and all of them as yet untested. Presentation of a variety of these techniques at conferences previously reserved for the more scientific exploration of PTSD has led to interest and excitement, as well as great controversy. At the same time, war, ethnic cleansing, tribal genocide, and natural disasters in Russia, Albania, Africa, Turkey, India, and Pakistan have continued to remind us of the inevitable presence of catastrophic trauma on our planet.

The theme of this book might appear to be overwhelmed by the enormity of the problem of pervasive life trauma, especially if one accepts the fact that even "trivial" trauma in childhood has lifelong implications. The other side of this discouraging coin, however, implies that simple attention to the role of these "trivial" traumatic life events may have disproportionately positive long-term effects. If we are able to conclude that many of the chronic, unexplained diseases that we treat so ineffectively may be based on a variation of autonomic dysregulation based on such cumulative life trauma, a whole new paradigm for prevention and management of these diseases may be developed.

In this perpetual and never-completed search for truth, I believe that one must combine the rigor and skepticism of the scientific with the wisdom and curiosity of the intuitive. Both approaches to the truth are subject to opportunism, bias, elitism, and financial secondary gain. But the blind application of science to the healing arts, by definition, limits our observations to the parameters for measurement that we have been able to standardize based on statistical limits that may miss the subtleties of clinical pathology. In this process of treading the fine line between art and science, the basic traditional diagnostic and intuitive skills of the physician-as-healer must never be allowed to fade and atrophy in the glare of technological advancement.

One must recognize that many legitimate techniques of the healing arts will never be adequately amenable to statistical validation by the scientific method. By the same token, diagnosis and treatment through intuitive techniques alone may open the way for opportunism and charlatanism. The only way that we may resolve this dilemma is for both sides of the issue—the intuitive and the scientific—to come together in recognition of the value of the other's position. Intuitive techniques, including untested somatically based trauma therapies, must be subjected to adequate, randomized controlled studies, and the scientific community responsible for funding of such rigorous studies must make a commitment to the more open process of investigation of novel, but compelling, therapies in the field of trauma.

Investigation of the role of brain development in the face of the subtleties of neglect must be pursued with open-minded but passionate intensity. Implication of neglect immediately casts a negative light on selected members of our society, and the pursuit of data in this area must be taken with compassion, understanding, and education. The rapidly evolving field of knowledge in the area of life trauma has opened a Pandora's box of information that has profound implications for the emotional and physical welfare of mankind. For the sake of mankind, further investigations in the field of the physiology of trauma and the nuances of its treatment must not be impeded by personal bias or political or professional self-interest.

Notes

Foreword

1. van der Kolk, B.A.: Post Traumatic Stress Disorder and the Nature of Trauma. *Dialogues in Clinical Neuroscience,* 2000, pp. 2, 7-22.
2. van der Kolk, B.A., McFarlane, A.C., and Weisaeth, L. (Eds.): *Traumatic stress: The effects of overwhelming experience on mind, body and society.* New York, Guilford Press, 1996.
3. Young, A.: *The Harmony of Illusions.* Oxford Universities Press, 1998.

Preface

1. *Stedman's Medical Dictionary:* Twenty-fourth Edition, Baltimore: Williams & Wilkins, 1982, p. 1382.
2. Levine, P.: *Waking the Tiger,* Berkeley, CA: North Atlantic Press, 1997.
3. Brown, T.: Cartesian dualism and psychosomatics, *Psychosomatics,* 1989; 30(3):322-331.
4. Descartes, R.: Meditation IV (1641). In *The Philosophical Works, Volume 1,* Translated by Haldane, E., Ross, D., New York/Dover, 1955, p. 2. In Brown, T.: Cartesian dualism and psychosomatics, *Psychosomatics,* 1989; 30(3):322-331, p. 325.
5. Descartes, R.: The Passions of the Soul (1649). In *The Philosophical Works, Volume 1,* translated by Haldane, E., Ross, D., New York/Dover, 1955, p. 2. In Brown, T.: Cartesian dualism and psychosomatics, *Psychosomatics,* 1989; 30:322-332, p. 325-326.

Chapter 1

1. American Psychiatric Association: *Diagnostic and Statistical Manual of Mental Disorders,* Fourth Edition (DSM-IV), Washington, DC: American Psychiatric Association, 1994.
2. American Psychiatric Association: *Diagnostic and Statistical Manual of Mental Disorders,* Third Edition (DSM-III), Washington, DC: American Psychiatric Association, 1981, p. 236.
3. Schore, A.: *Affect Regulation and the Origin of the Self,* Hillsdale, NJ: Lawrence Erlbaum Associates, 1994.

Chapter 2

1. Cannon, W.: The emergency function of the adrenal medulla and the major emotions, *American Journal of Physiology,* 1914; 33:356-372.

2. Selye, H.: *The Stress of Life,* New York: McGraw-Hill, 1956.

3. LeDoux, J.: *Mind and Brain: Dialogues in Cognitive Neuroscience,* New York: Cambridge University Press, 1986.

4. van der Kolk, B.: The body keeps the score: Memory and the evolving psychobiology of posttraumatic stress, *Harvard Review of Psychiatry,* 1994;1(5): 253-265.

5. Levine, P.: Stress, in Coles, M., Donchin, E., Porges, S., Eds., *Psychophysiology,* New York: The Guilford Press, 1986.

6. Mason, J.: Confusion and controversy in the stress field, *Journal of Human Stress,* 1975;1:6-35.

7. van der Kolk, B., Greenberg, M., Orr, S., Pitman, R.: Endogenous opioids and stress-induced analgesia in posttraumatic stress disorder, *Psychopharmacological Bulletin,* 1989; 25:108-112.

8. Pitman, R., van der Kolk, B., Orr, S., Greenberg, M.: Naloxone reversible stress-induced analgesia in posttraumatic stress disorder, *Archives of General Psychiatry,* 1990; 47:541-547.

9. Hess, W.: *Das Zwischenhirn,* Basel: Schwabe, 1949.

10. Mc Gaugh, J.: Involvement of hormonal and neuromodulatory systems in the regulation of memory storage, *Annual Review of Neuroscience,* 1989; 2:255-287.

11. Seligman, M.E.P., Maier, S.F.: Failure to escape traumatic shock, *Journal of Experimental Psychology,* 1967; 74:1-9.

12. Seligman, M.W.D.: *Helplessness: On Depression, Development and Death,* San Francisco: Freeman, 1975.

13. Bouton, M.C., Bolles, R.C.: Conditioned fear assessed by freezing and by the suppression of three different baselines, *Animal Learning and Behavior,* 1980; 429-434.

14. Fanselow, M.S., Lester, L.S.: A functional behavioristic approach to aversively motivated behavior: Predatory imminence as a determinant of the topography of defensive behavior. In Bolles, R.C., Beecher, M.D., Eds., *Evolution and Learning,* Hillsdale, NJ: Lawrence Erlbaum Associates, 1988, pp. 185-212.

15. van der Kolk, B.A., Greenberg, M.S., Boyd, H., Krystal, J.: Inescapable shock, neurotransmitters and addiction to trauma: Towards a psychobiology of posttraumatic stress, *Biologic Psychiatry,* 1985; 20:314-325.

16. Nijenhuis, E.R.S., Venderlinden, J., Spinhoven, P.: *Journal of Traumatic Stress,* 1998; 11(2):243-260.

17. Gellhorn, E.: The tuning of the autonomic nervous system through the alteration of the internal environment (asphyxia), *Acta Neurologica,* 1960; 20:515-540.

18. Levine, P.: *Waking the Tiger,* Berkeley, CA: North Atlantic Press, 1997.

19. *Stedman's Medical Dictionary:* Twenty-fourth Edition, Baltimore: Williams & Wilkins, 1982, p. 416.

Chapter 3

1. Trimble, M.: *Post-Traumatic Neurosis,* Chichester, England: John Wiley & Sons, 1981.

2. Marshall, H.: Neck injuries, *Boston Medical Surgical Journal,* 1919; 180:93-98.

3. Davis, A.: Injuries of the cervical spine, *JAMA,* 1945;127:149-156.

4. Gay, J., Abbott, K.: Common whiplash injuries of the neck, *JAMA,* 1953; 152:1699.

5. Severy, D., Mathewson, J., Bechtol, C.: Controlled automobile rear-end collisions, and investigation of related engineering and medical phenomena, *Canadian Services Medical Journal,* 1955;11:728.

6. Allen, M., Weir-Jones, I., Eng, P., Motiuk, D., Flewin, K., Goring, R., Kobetitch, R., Broadhurst, A.: Acceleration perturbations of daily living: A comparison to "whiplash," *Spine,* 1994; 19(11):1285-1290.

7. Bosworth, D.: (Editorial) *Journal of Bone and Joint Surgery,* 1959; 41-A:16.

8. Radanov, P., DiStefano, G., Schindrig, A., Ballinari, P.: The role of psychosocial stress in recovery from common whiplash, *Lancet,* 1991; 338:712-715.

9. Balla, J.: Report to the Motor Accident Board of Victoria on whiplash injuries, 1984. In Hopkins, A. Ed., Headache, problems in diagnosis and management, (pp. 256-269) *Headache and Cervical Disorders,* London: Saunders, 1988.

10. Pearce, J.: Whiplash injury: A reappraisal, *Journal of Neurology and Neurosurgery,* 1989; 52:1329-1331.

11. Friedmann, L., Marin, E., Padula, P.: Biomechanics of cervical trauma. In Tollison, C., Satterthwaite, J. Eds., *Painful Cervical Trauma: Diagnosis and Rehabilitative Treatment of Neuromuscular Injuries* (pp. 10-19), 1992.

12. Packard, R., Ham, L.: Posttraumatic headache, *Journal of Neuropsychiatry,* 1994; 6:119-136.

13. McNab, I.: The whiplash syndrome, *Orthopedic Clinics of North America,* 1971; 2:389-403.

14. Luo, Z., Goldsmith, W.: Reaction of a human head/neck/torso system to shock, *Journal of Biomechanics,* 1991; 24(7):499-510.

15. McConnell, W., Howark R., Guzman, H., Bomar, J., Raddian, J., Benedict, V., Smith, H., and Hatsell, C.: Analysis of human test subject kinematic responses to low velocity rear end impacts, 1993; Society of Automotive Engineers 930899.

16. Pettersson, K., Hildingsson, C., Toolanen, S., Fagerlund, M., Bjornebrink, J.: MRI and neurology in acute whiplash trauma, *Acta Orthopedica Scandinavia,* 1994; 65:525-528.

17. Ommaya, A., Faas, F., Yarnell, P.: Whiplash injury and brain damage—an experimental study, *JAMA,* 1968; 204:285-289.

18. Weinberg, S., LaPointe, H.: Cervical extension-flexion injury (whiplash) and internal derangement of the temporomandibular joint, *Journal of Oral and Maxillofacial Surgery,* 1987; 45:653-659.

19. Wickstrom, J., Martinez, J., Rodriguez, T.: Cervical sprain syndrome and experimental acceleration injuries of the head and neck. In Selzer, M., Gikas, P.,

Huelke, P., Eds., *Proceedings of Prevention of Highway Accidents Symposium* (pp. 182-187), Ann Arbor, MI: University of Michigan, 1967.

20. Oosterveld, W., Kortschot, H., Kingma, G., de Jong, H., Saatsi, M.: Electronystagmographic findings following cervical whiplash injuries, *Acta Otolaryngol*, (Stockholm) 1991; 111:201-205.

21. Roy, R.: The role of binocular stress in the post-whiplash syndrome, *American Journal of Optometry and Archives of American Academy of Optometry*, November 1961; 1-11.

22. Helleday, U.: Om mysitis chronica (rheumatica). Ett bidrag till dess diagnostik och behandling, *Mord Med Ark*, 1876; 8:art 8.

23. Gowers, W.: A lecture on lumbago: Its lessons and analogues, *British Medical Journal*, 1904; 1:117-121.

24. Peritz, G.: *Med Klinik*, 1906; 2:1145.

25. Travell, J., Rinzler, S.: The myofascial genesis of pain. *Postgraduate Medicine*, 1952; 11:425-434.

26. Travell, J., Simons, D.: *Myofascial Pain and Dysfunction: The Trigger Point Manual*, Baltimore: Williams & Wilkins, 1983.

27. Simons, D.: Clinical features of myofascial trigger points, *Journal of Musculoskeletal Pain*, 1996; 4(1,2):95-121.

28. Hubbard, D.: Chronic and recurrent muscle pain: Pathophysiology and treatment, and review of pharmacological studies, *Journal of Musculoskeletal Pain*, 1996; 4(1,1,2):123-143.

29. Hong, C., Simons, S.: Pathophysiologic and electrophysiologic mechanisms of myofascial trigger points, *Archives of Physical Medicine and Rehabilitation*, 998; 79:863-871.

30. Donaldson, C., Nelson, D., Schulz, R.: Disinihibition in the gamma motoneuron circuitry: A neglected mechanism for understanding myofascial pain syndrome? *Applied Psychophysiology and Biofeedback*, 1998; 23(1):43-57.

31. Elson, L.: The jolt syndrome: Muscle dysfunction following low-velocity impact, *Pain Management*, 1990; November/December: 317-326.

32. Ellison, D., Wood, V.: Trauma-related thoracic outlet syndrome, *Journal of Hand Surgery*, 1994; 19B:424-426.

33. Lader, E.: Cervical trauma as a factor in the development of TMJ dysfunction and facial pain, *Journal of Craniomandibular Practice*, 1983; 1:88-90.

34. Levandoski, R.: Mandibular whiplash, Part 1: An extension/flexion injury of the temporomandibular joints, *The Functional Orthodontist*, 1993; January/February:26-33.

35. Mild Traumatic Brain Injury Committee of the Interdisciplinary Special Interest Group of the American Congress of Rehabilitation Medicine, in *The Journal of Head Trauma Rehabilitation*, 1993; 8:3:86-88.

36. Jane, J., Steward, O., Gennarelli, T.: Axonal degeneration induced by experimental noninvasive minor head injury, *Journal of Neurosurgery*, 1985; 62:96-100.

37. Povlishock, J., Becker, D., Cheng, C., Vaughan, G.: Axonal change in minor head injury, *Journal of Neuropathology and Experimental Neurology,* 1983; 42: 225-242.

38. Gronwall, D., Wrightson, P.: Memory and information processing capacity after closed head injury, *Journal of Neurology, Neurosurgery, and Psychiatry,* 1981; 44:889-895.

39. Stuss, D., Stethem, L., Hugenholtz, H., Picton, T., Pivik, J., Richard, M.: Reaction time after head injury: Fatigue, divided and focused attention, and consistency of performance, *Journal of Neurology, Neurosurgery and Psychiatry,*1989: 52:742-748.

40. Gentilini, M., Nichelli, P., Schoenhuber, R., Bartolotti, P., Tonelli, L., Falasca, A., Merli, G.: Assessment of attention in mild head injury. In Levin, H., Eisenberg, H., Benton, A., Eds: *Mild Head Injury* (pp. 163-175), New York: Oxford University Press, 1989.

41. Binder, L.: Persisting symptoms after mild head injury: A review of the postconcussive syndrome, *Journal of Clinical and Experimental Neuropsychology,* 1986; 8:323-346.

42. Boquet, J., Moore, N., Boismare, F., Monnier, J.: Vertigo in postconcussional and migrainous patients: Implication of the autonomic nervous system, *Agressologie,* 1983; 24:235-236.

43. Grimm, R., Hemenway, W., Sebray, P., Black, F.: The perilymph fistula syndrome defined in mild head trauma, *Acta Otolaryngol* (Stockholm) 1989; 262(supplement):1-40.

44. Blanchard, W., Hickling, E.: *After the Crash,* Washington, DC: American Psychological Association Press, 1997.

45. Miller, H.: Accident neurosis, *British Medical Journal,* 1961; 1:919-925; 992-998.

46. Alexander, M.: Neuropsychiatric correlates of persistent postconcussive syndrome, *Journal of Head Trauma Rehabilitation,* 1992; 7(2):60-69.

Chapter 4

1. van der Kolk, B., van der Hart, O.: The intrusive past: The flexibility of memory and the engraving of trauma, *American Imago,* 1991; 48:425-454.

2. van der Kolk, B.: The body keeps the score: Memory and the evolving psychobiology of posttraumatic stress, *Harvard Review of Psychiatry,* 1994; 1(5): 253-265.

3. McGaugh, J., Weinberger, N., Lynch, G., Granger, R.: Neural mechanisms of learning and memory: Cells, systems, and computations, *Naval Reserve Review,* 1989; 37:15-29.

4. Roediger, H.: Implicit memory: Retention without remembering, *American Psychologist,* 1990; 45:1043-1056.

5. Squire, L., Zola-Morgan, S.: The medial temporal lobe memory system, *Science,* 1991; 253:2380-2385.

6. Altman, J., Brunner, R., Bayer, S.: The hippocampus and behavioral maturation, *Behavioral Biology,* 1973; 8:557-596.

7. Duffy, C.: Implicit memory: Knowledge without awareness, *Neurology,* 1997; 49:1200-1202.

8. Sturtzenetter, N., DiStafano, G., Radanov, B., Schnidrig, A.: Presenting symptoms and signs after whiplash injury: The influence of accident mechanisms, *Neurology,* 1994; 44:688-693.

9. Trimble, M.: *Post-Traumatic neurosis,* Chichester, England: John Wiley & Sons, 1981.

10. Goddard, G., McIntyre, D., Leetch C.: A permanent change in brain functioning resulting from daily electrical stimulation, *Experimental Neurology,* 1969; 25: 295-330.

11. Post, R., Weiss, S., Smith, M.: Sensitization and kindling: Implications for the evolving neural substrate of post-traumatic stress disorder. In Friedman, M., Charney, D., Deutch, A., Eds., *Neurobiological and Clinical Consequences of Stress: From Normal Adaptation to PTSD* (pp. 203-224), Philadelphia: Lippincott-Raven Publishers: 1995.

12. Miller, L.: Neurosensitization: A pathophysiological model for traumatic disability syndromes, *The Journal of Cognitive Rehabilitation,* 1997;12-23.

13. Charney, D., Deutsch, A., Krystal, J., Southwick, S., Davis, M.: Psychobiologic mechanisms of posttraumatic stress disorder, *Archives of General Psychiatry,* 1993; 50: 294-305.

14. Blanchard, E., Hickling, E.: *After the Crash,* Washington, DC: American Psychological Association Press, 1997.

15. Bremner, D., Scott, T., Delaney, R., Southwick, S., Mason, J., Johnson, D., Innis, J., McCarthy, G., Charney, D.: Deficits in short-term memory in posttraumatic stress disorder, *American Journal of Psychiatry,* 1993; 150(7):1015-1019.

16. Alexander, M.: Neuropsychiatric correlates of persistent postconcussive syndrome, *Journal of Head Trauma Rehabilitation,* 1992; 7(2):60-69.

17. Gill, T., Calev, A., Greenberg, D., Kugelmas, S., Lerer, B.: Cognitive functioning in posttraumatic stress disorder, *Journal of Traumatic Stress,* 1990; 3:29-45.

18. Miller, L.: The "trauma" of head trauma: Clinical, neuropsychological and forensic aspects of chemical and electrical injuries, *Journal of Cognitive Rehabilitation,* 1993; 11(4):6-18.

19. Weiner, H.: *Perturbing the Organism: The Biology of the Stressful Experience,* Chicago: University of Chicago Press, 1992.

20. Siegfried, B., Frischknecht, H., Nunez de Souza, T.: An ethological model for the study of activation and interaction of pain, memory, and defensive systems in the attacked mouse: Role of endogenous opioids. *Neuroscience Biobehavioral Review,* 1990; 14:481-490.

21. Sapolsky, R., Uno, H., Rebert, C., Finch, C.: Hippocampal damage with prolonged glucocorticoid exposure in primates, *The Journal of Neuroscience,* 1990; 10(9): 2897-2902.

22. Sapolsky, R., Packan, D., Vale, W.: Glucocorticoid toxicity in the hippocampus: In vitro demonstration, *Brain Research,* 1988; 453:367-371.

23. Uno, H., Tarara, R., Else, J., Suleman, M., Sapolsky, R.: Hippocampal damage associated with prolonged and fatal stress in primates, *The Journal of Neuroscience,* 1989; 9(5):1705-1711.

24. Beecher, H.: Pain in men wounded in battle, *Annals of Surgery,* 1946; 123:95-105.

25. Machuda, M., Bergquist, T., Ito, V., Chew, S.: Relationship between stress, coping, and postconcussion symptoms in a healthy adult population, *Archives of Clinical Neuropsychology,* 1998; 13(5):415-424.

26. Shalev, A.Y., Rogel-Fuchs, Y.: Psychophysiology of the posttraumatic stress disorder: From sulfur fumes to behavioral genetics, *Psychosomatic Medicine,* 1993; 55:413-423.

27. Evans, R.W.: Some observations on whiplash injuries, *Neurologic Clinics,* 1992; 10(4):975-996.

28. LeDoux, J., Romanski, L., Xagoras, A.: Indelibility of subcortical emotional memories, *Journal of Cognitive Neuroscience,* 1989; 1(3):238-243.

Chapter 5

1. van der Kolk, B., Weisaeth, L., van der Hart, O.: The history of trauma in psychiatry. In van der Kolk, B., McFarlane, A., Weisaeth, L., Eds., *Traumatic Stress,* New York: The Guilford Press, 1996.

2. Noyes, A., Kolb, L.: *Modern Clinical Psychiatry,* Philadelphia: W.B. Saunders Company, 1958.

3. Janet, P.: *L'automatisme Psychologique,* Paris: Alcan, 1889.

4. van der Kolk, B., van der Hart, O.: Pierre Janet and the breakdown of adaptation in psychological trauma, *Journal of Psychiatry,* 1989; 146:1520-1540.

5. Freud, S.: The aetiology of hysteria. In Strachey, J., Ed. and Trans., *The Standard Edition of the Complete Psychological Works of Sigmund Freud* (Volume 15, pp.1-240; Volume 16, pp. 241-496). London: Hogarth Press. (Original work published 1896).

6. Miller, A.: *Banished Knowledge: Facing Childhood Injuries,* New York: Anchor Books, Doubleday, 1990.

7. Freud, S.: The interpretation of dreams. In Strachey, J. Ed. and Trans., *The Standard Edition of the Complete Psychological Works of Sigmund Freud* (Volume 7, pp. 125-243). London: Hogarth Press. (Original work published 1905).

8. Kardiner, A.: *The Traumatic Neuroses of War,* New York: Hoeber, 1941.

9. Eitinger, L., Strom, A.: *Mortality and Morbidity After Excessive Stress: A Follow-Up Investigation of Norwegian Concentration Camp Survivors,* Oslo: Universitetsforlaget, 1973.

10. Hocking, F.: Psychiatric aspects of extreme environmental stress, *Diseases of the Nervous System,* 1970; 31:1278-1282.

11. Burgess, A., Holstrom, L.: Rape trauma syndrome, *American Journal of Psychiatry,* 1974; 131:981-986.

12. Kempe, R., Kempe, C.: *Child Abuse,* Cambridge, MA: Harvard University Press, 1978.

13. van der Kolk, B., Greenberg, M., Boyd, H., Krystal, J.: Inescapable shock, neurotransmitters and addiction to trauma: Toward a psychobiology of post-traumatic stress disorder, *Biological Psychiatry,* 1985; 20:314-325.

14. Schore, A.: *Affect Regulation and the Origin of the Self,* Hillsdale, NJ: Lawrence Erlbaum Associates, 1994.

15. Hofer, M.: Early symbiotic processes: Hard evidence from a soft place. In Glick, R., Bone, S., Eds., *Pleasure Beyond the Pleasure Principle* (pp. 55-78), New Haven: Yale University Press, 1990.

16. Mattson, M.: Neurotransmitters in the regulation of neuronal cytoarchitecture, *Brain Research Review,* 1988; 13:179-212.

17. Schore, A.: The experience-dependent maturation of a regulatory system in the orbital pre-frontal cortex and the origin of developmental psychopathology, *Development and Psychopathology,* 1996; 8:59-87.

18. Greenough, W.: What's special about development? Thoughts on the bases of experience-sensitive synaptic plasticity. In Greenough, W., Juraska, J. Eds., *Developmental Neuropsychology,* New York: Academic Press, 1986, pp. 387-407.

19. Hubel, D., Wiesel, T.: Receptive fields of cells in striate cortex of very young, visually inexperienced kittens, *Journal of Neurophysiology,* 1963; 26:994-1009.

20. Hubel, D., Wiesel, T., LeVay, S.: Plasticity of ocular dominance columns in monkey striate cortex, *Philosophical Transactions of the Royal Society of London,* 1977; B:278:377-409.

21. Grigsby, J., Hartlaub, G.: Procedural learning and the development and stability of character, *Perceptual and Motor Skills,* 1994; 79:355-370.

22. Gazzaniga, M.: *The Social Brain,* New York: Basic Books, 1985.

23. van der Kolk, B.: The body keeps the score: Memory and the evolving psychobiology of posttraumatic stress, *Harvard Review of Psychiatry,* 1994; 1: 253-265.

24. Grigsby, J.: Combat rush: Phenomenology of central and autonomic arousal among war veterans with PTSD, *Psychotherapy,* 1991; 28:354-363.

25. Shalev, A., Rogel-Fuchs, M.: Psychophysiology of the posttraumatic stress disorder: From sulfur fumes to behavioral genetics, *Psychosomatic Medicine,* 1993; 55:413-423.

26. Kolb, L.: A neurophysiological hypothesis explaining the posttraumatic stress disorder, *American Journal of Psychiatry,* 1987; 144:989-995.

27. Blanchard, B., Hickling, E., Taylor, A.: The psychophysiology of motor vehicle accident related posttraumatic stress disorder, *Biofeedback and Self-Regulation,* 1991; 16(4):449-458.

28. Pavlov, I.: *Conditioned reflexes: An investigation of the physiological activity of the cerebral cortex,* (1927); Edited and translated by Anrep, G.V., New York: Dover, 1960.

29. Keane, T., Kaloupek, D.: Imaginal flooding in the treatment of a posttraumatic stress disorder, *Journal of Consulting and Clinical Psychology,* 1982; 50:138-140.

30. Bremner, J., Scott, M., Delaney, T., Southwick, S., Mason, J., Johnson, D., Innis, T., McCarthy, G., Charney, D.: Deficits in short-term memory in posttraumatic stress disorder, *American Journal of Psychiatry,* 1993; 150:1015-1019.

31. Bremner, J., Randall, P., Scott, T., Bronen, R., Seibyl, J., Southwick, S., Delaney, R., McCarthy, G., Charney, D., Innis, R.: MRI-based measures of hippocampal volume in patients with PTSD, *American Journal of Psychiatry,* 1995; 152:973-981.

32. Stein, M., Hannah, C., Koverola, C., Yehuda, R., Torchia, M., McClarty, B.: Neuroanatomical and neuroendocrine correlates in adulthood of severe sexual abuse in childhood. Presented at the thirty-third annual meeting of the American College of Neuropsychopharmacology, San Juan, PR, 1994.

33. Sapolsky, R., Packan, D., Vale, W.: Glucocorticoid toxicity in the hippocampus: In vitro demonstration, *Brain Research,* 1988; 453:367-371.

34. Sapolsky, R., Uno, H., Rebert, C., Finch, C.: Hippocampal damage associated with prolonged glucocorticoid exposure in primates, *Journal of Neuroscience,* 1990; 10(9):2897-2902.

35. Uno, H., Tarara, R., Else, J., Suleman, M., Sapolsky, R.: Hippocampal damage associated with prolonged and fatal stress in primates, *Journal of Neuroscience,* 1989; 9(5):1705-1711.

36. Rauch, S., van der Kolk, B., Fisler, R., Alpert, N., Orr, S., Savage, C., Fischman, A., Jenike, M., Pitman, R.: A symptom provocation study of posttraumatic stress disorder using positron emission tomography and script-driven imagery, *Archives of General Psychiatry,* 1996; 53:380-387.

37. Shin, L., McNally, R., Kosslyn, S., Thompson, W., Rauch, S., Alpert, N., Metzger, L., Lasko, N., Orr., S., Pitman, T.: Regional cerebral blood flow during script-driven imagery in childhood sexual abuse-related PTSD: A PET investigation, *American Journal of Psychiatry,* 1999; 156(4):575-584.

38. Bremner, J.: Alterations in brain structure and function associated with posttraumatic stress disorder, *Seminars in Clinical Neuropsychiatry,* 1999; 4(4): 249-255.

39. Tichener, J.: Post-traumatic decline: A consequence of unresolved destructive drives. In Figley, C., Ed., *Trauma and its Wake* (Volume 2, pp. 5-19), New York: Brunner-Mazel, 1986.

40. Mason, J., Giller, E., Kosten, T., Ostroff, R., Podd, L.: Urinary free-cortisol levels in posttraumatic stress disorder patients, *Journal of Nervous and Mental Disease,* 1986; 174(3):145-149.

41. Mason, J., Giller, E., Kosten, T., Harkness, L.: Elevation of urinary norepinephrine/cortisol ratio in posttraumatic stress disorder, 1988; 176(8):498-502.

42. Friedman, S., Mason, J., Hamburg, D.: Urinary 17-hydroxycorticosteroid levels in parents of children with neoplastic disease, *Psychosomatic Medicine,* 1963; 25:364-376.

43. Mason, J.: Clinical psychophysiology: Psychoendocrine mechanisms. In Reiser, M., Ed., *American Handbook of Psychiatry* (Volume 4, pp. 553-582), New York: Basic Books, 1975.

44. Shalev, A., Peri, T., Caneti, L., Schreiber, S.: Predictors of PTSD in injured trauma survivors: A prospective study, *American Journal of Psychiatry*, 1996; 153: 219-225.

45. van der Kolk, B., Greenburg, M., Orr, S., Pitman, R.: Endogenous opioids and stress-induced analgesia in posttraumatic stress disorder, *Psychopharmacology Bulletin*, 1989; 25:108-112.

Chapter 6

1. Selye, H.: Thymus and adrenals in the response of the organism to injuries and intoxications, *British Journal of Experimental Pathology*, 1936; 17:234-246.

2. Mason, J., Giller, E., Kosten, T., Ostroff, R., Podd, L.: Urinary-free cortisol levels in posttraumatic stress disorder patients, *Journal of Nervous and Mental Disease*,1986; 174(3):145-159.

3. Yehuda, R., Boisoneau, D., Mason, J., Giller, E.: Relationship between lymphocyte glucocorticoid receptor number and urinary-free cortisol excretion in mood, anxiety, and psychotic disorders, *Biological Psychiatry*, 1993; 34:18-25.

4. Yehuda, R., Southwick, S., Nussbaum, G., Giller, E., Mason, J.: Low urinary cortisol excretion in PTSD, *Journal of Nervous and Mental Disease*, 1991; 178: 366-369.

5. Yehuda, R., Giller, E., Southwick, S., Lowy, M., Mason, J.: Hypothalamic-pituitary-adrenal dysfunction in posttraumatic stress disorder, *Biological Psychiatry*, 1993; 30:1031-1048.

6. Breslau, N., Davis, G., Andreski, P., Peterson, E.: Traumatic events and posttraumatic stress disorder in an urban population of young adults, *Archives of General Psychiatry*, 1991; 48:216-222.

7. Yehuda, R., Giller, W., Levengood, R., Southwick, S., Siever, L.: Hypothalamic-pituitary-adrenal functioning in post-traumatic stress disorder. In Friedman, M., Charney, D., Deutch, A., Eds., *Neurobiologic and Clinical Consequences of Stress: From Normal to PTSD* (pp. 351-365), Philadelphia: Lippincott-Raven Publishers.

8. Cohen, S., Tyrrell, D., Smith, S.: Psychological stress and susceptibility to the common cold, *New England Journal of Medicine*, 1991: 325:606-612.

9. Petry, L., Weems, L., Livingstone, J.: Relationship of stress, distress, and the immunologic response to a recombinant Hepatitis B vaccine, *Journal of Family Practice*, 1991; 32:481-486.

10. Keicolt-Glaser, J., Fisher, L., Ogrocki, P., Stout, J., Speicher, C., Glaser, R.: Marital quality, marital disruption, and immune function, *Psychosomatic Medicine*, 1987; 49:13-34.

11. McKinnon, W., Weisse, C., Reynolds, C., Bowles, C., Baum, A.: Chronic stress, leukocyte subpopulations, and humoral response to latent viruses, *Health Psychology*, 1989; 8:389-401.

12. Goodkin, K., Fuchs, I., Feaster, D., Leeka, J., Rishel, D.: Life stressors and coping style are associated with immune measures in HIV-1 infection—a preliminary report, *International Journal of Psychiatry and Medicine*, 1992; 22:155-172.

13. Ironside, G., LaPerriere, A., Antoni, M., O'Hearn, J., Schneiderman, N., Klimas, N., Fletcher, M.: Changes in immune and psychological measures as a function of anticipation and reaction to news of HIV-1 antibody status, *Psychosomatic Medicine,* 1990; 52:247-270.

14. Benschop, R., Niewenhuis, E., Tromp, E., Godaert, G., Ballieux, R., Vandoornen, L.: Effects of beta-adrenergic blockade on immunologic and cardiovascular changes induced by mental stress, *Circulation,* 1994; 89:762-769.

15. Knudsen, J., Kjaersgaard, E., Jensen, E., Christensen, N.: Percentage of NK-cells in peripheral blood in resting normal subjects is negatively correlated to plasma adrenaline, *Scandinavian Journal of Clinical Laboratory Investigation,* 1994; l54:221-225.

16. Benschop, R., Broschot, J., Godaert, G., DeSmet, M., Geenen, R., Olff, M., Heijnen, C., Ballieux, R.: Chronic stress affects immunologic but not cardiovascular responsiveness to acute psychological stress in humans, *American Journal of Physiology,* 1994; 266:R75-R80.

17. Finkelhor, D.: *Sexually Victimized Children,* New York: Free Press, 1979.

18. Kirkpatrick, D., Edmunds, C.: *Rape in America: A Report to the Nation,* Arlington, VA: National Victim Center, Charleston, SC, Crime Victims Research and Treatment Center, April, 1992.

19. Rowan, A., Foy, D.: Post-traumatic stress disorder in child sexual abuse survivors: A literature review, *Journal of Traumatic Stress,* 1993; 6:3.

20. Springs, F., Friedrich, W.: Health risk behaviors and medical sequelae of childhood sexual abuse, *Mayo Clinic Proceedings,* 1992; 67:527.

21. Fromuth, M., Burkhart, B.: Long-term psychological correlates of childhood sexual abuse in two samples of college men, *Child Abuse and Neglect,* 1989; 13:533.

22. Courtois, C.: Adult survivors of sexual abuse, *Primary Care,* 1993; 20:433.

23. Bolen, J.: The impact of sexual abuse on women's health, *Psychiatric Annals,* 1993; 23:446.

24. Walker, E., Katon, W., Harrop-Griffiths, J., Holm, L., Russo, J., Hickock, L.: Relationship of chronic pelvic pain to psychiatric diagnosis and childhood sexual abuse, *American Journal of Psychiatry,* 1988; 145:75-80.

25. Reiter, D.: The incidence and prevalence of women with chronic pelvic pain, *Clinical Obstetrics and Gynecology,* 1990; 33:130-136.

26. Toomey, T., Hernandez, J., Gittelman, K., Hulka, J.: Relationship of sexual and physical abuse to pain and psychological assessment variables in chronic pelvic pain patients, *Pain,* 1993; 53:105-109.

27. Walling, M., Reiter, R., O'Hara, M., Milburn, A., Lilly, G., Vincent, S.: Abuse history and chronic pain in women: I. Prevalence of sexual abuse and physical abuse, *Obstetrics and Gynecology,* 1994; 84:193-199.

28. Walker, E., Katon, W., Hansom, J., Harrops-Griffiths, J., Holm, L., Jones, M., Hickock, L., Jemelka, R.: Medical and psychiatric symptoms in women with childhood sexual abuse, *Psychosomatic Medicine,* 1992; 54:638-664.

29. Rapkin, A., Kames, L., Darke, L., Stampler, F., Nabiloff, B.: History of physical and sexual abuse in women with chronic pelvic pain, *Obstetrics and Gynecology,* 1990; 76:92-96.

30. Walling, M., O'Hara, M., Reiter, R., Milburn, A., Lilly, G., Vincent, S.: Abuse history and chronic pain in women: II. A multivariate analysis of abuse and psychological morbidity, *Obstetrics and Gynecology,* 1994; 84(2):200-206.

31. Curran, S., Sherman, J., Cunningham, L., Okeson, J., Reid, K., Carlson, S.: Physical and sexual abuse among orofacial pain patients: Linkages with pain and psychologic distress, *Journal of Orofacial Pain,* 1995; 9(4):340-344.

32. Woods, D.: Sexual abuse during childhood and adolescence and its effects on the physical and emotional quality of life of the survivor: A review of the literature, *Military Medicine,* 1996; 161:582-587.

33. Wurtele, S., Kaplan, G., Keairnes, M.: Childhood sexual abuse among chronic pain patients, *The Clinical Journal of Pain,* 1990; 6:110-113.

34. Schofferman, J., Anderson, D., Hines, R., Smith, G., Keane, G.: Childhood psychological trauma and chronic refractory low-back pain, *The Clinical Journal of Pain,* 1993; 9:260-329.

35. Goldberg, R.: Childhood abuse, depression, and chronic pain, *The Clinical Journal of Pain,* 1994; 10:277-281.

36. Mitchell, S., Morehouse, G., Keen, W.: *Gunshot Wounds and Other Injuries,* Philadelphia: J.B. Lippincott Co., 1864.

37. Escobar, P.: Reflex sympathetic dystrophy, *Orthopedic Review,* 1986; 15:646.

38. Schwartzman, R., McLellan, T.: Reflex sympathetic dystrophy: A review, *Archives of Neurology,* 1987; 44:555.

39. Steinbroker, O.: The shoulder-hand syndrome, *American Journal of Medicine,* 1947; 3:403.

40. Lankford, L.: Reflex sympathetic dystrophy. In Omer, G., Spinner, M., Eds., *Management of Peripheral Nerve Problems* (pp. 216-244), Philadelphia: Saunders, 1980.

41. Khurana, R., Nirankari, V.: Bilateral sympathetic dysfunction in post-traumatic headaches, *Headache,* 1986; April:183-188.

42. Gowers, W.: Lumbago: Its lessons and analogues, *British Medical Journal,* 1904; 1:117-121.

43. Moldofsky, H.: Sleep and musculoskeletal pain, *American Journal of Medicine,* 1986; 81(Supplement 3A):85-89.

44. Waylonis, G., Perkins, R.: Post-traumatic fibromyalgia: A long-term follow-up, *American Journal of Physical Medicine and Rehabilitation,* 1994; 73(6):403-412.

45. Crofford, L.: The hypothalamic-pituitary-adrenal stress axis in the fibromyalgia syndrome, *Journal of Musculoskeletal Pain,* 1996; 4(1/2):181-200.

46. Demitrack, M., Dale, J., Strauss, S., Laue, L., Listwak, S., Kruesi, M., Chrousos, G., Gold, P.: Evidence for impaired activation of the hypothalamic-pituitary-adrenal axis in patients with chronic fatigue syndrome, *Journal of Clinical Endocrine Metabolism,* 1991; 73:1224-1234.

47. Bennett, R., Cook, D., Clark , S., Burckhardt, C., Campbell, S.: Hypothalamic-pituitary-insulin-like growth factor-I axis dysfunction in patients with fibromyalgia, *Journal of Rheumatology,* 1997; 24(7):1384-1388.

48. Rollman, G., Lautenbaacher, S.: Hypervigilence effects in fibromyalgia: Pain experience and pain perception. In Vaeroy, H., Merskey, H. Eds., *Progress in Fibromyalgia and Myfascial Pain* (pp. 149-159), Amsterdam: Elsevier: 1993.

49. McDermid, A., Rollman, G., McCain, G.: Generalized hypervigilance in fibromyalgia: Evidence of perceptual amplification, *Pain,* 1996; 66:133-144.

50. Taylor, M., Trotter, D., Csuka, M.: The prevalence of sexual abuse in women with fibromyalgia, *Arthritis and Rheumatism,* 1995; 38(2):229-234.

51. Boisset-Pioro, M., Esdaile, J., Fitzcharles, M.: Sexual and physical abuse in women with fibromyalgia syndrome, *Arthritis and Rheumatism,* 1995; 38(2): 235-241.

52. Rimsza, M., Berg, R.: Sexual abuse: Somatic and emotional reactions, *Child Abuse and Neglect,* 1988; 12:201-208.

53. Drossman, D., Leserman, J., Nachman, G., Li, X., Gluck, H., Toomey, T., Mitchell, M.: Sexual and physical abuse in women with functional or organic gastrointestinal disorders, *Annals of Internal Medicine,* 1990; 113(11):828-833.

54. Bachman, G., Moeller, T., Bennett, J.: Childhood sexual abuse and the consequence in adult women, *Obstetrics and Gynecology,* 1088; 71:631-642.

55. Friedman, M., Schnurr, P.: The relationship between trauma, post-traumatic stress disorder, and physical health. In Friedman, M., Charney, D., Deutch, A., Eds., *Neurobiological and Clinical Consequences of Stress: From Normal Adaptation to PTSD* (pp. 518-524), Philadelphia: Lippincott-Raven Publishers, 1995.

56. Beebe, G.: Followup studies of World War II and Korean War prisoners: II. Morbidity, disability, and maladjustments, *American Journal of Epidemiology,* 1975; 101:400-422.

57. Page, W.: *The Health of Former Prisoners of War,* Washington, DC: National Academy Press, 1992.

58. Cohen, B., Cooper, M.: *A Follow-Up Study of World War II Prisoners of War.* (Veterans Administration Medical Monograph). Washington, DC: Government Printing Office, 1955.

59. Sibi, A., Armenian, H., Alam, S.: Wartime determinants of arteriographically confirmed coronary artery disease in Beirut, *American Journal of Epidemiology,* 1989; 130:623-631.

60. Bergovec, M., Mihatov, S., Prpic, H., Rogan, S., Batarelo, V., Sjerobabski, V.: Acute myocardial infarction among civilians in Zagreb city area, *Lancet,* 1992; 339:303.

61. Felitti, V., Anda, T., Nordenberg, D., Williamson, D., Spitz, A., Edwards, V., Koss, M., Marks, J.: Relationship of childhood abuse and household dysfunction to many of the leading causes of death in adults: The adverse childhood experiences (ACE) study, *American Journal of Preventive Medicine,* 1998; 14(4):245-257.

62. Wolff, J., Schnurr, P., Brown, P., Furey, J.: PTSD and war-zone exposure as correlates of perceived health in female Vietnam veterans, *Journal of Consulting Clinical Psychology,* 1994; 62:1235-1240.

63. Falger, P., Op den Velde, W., Hovens, J., Schouten, E., DeGroen, J., Van Kuijn, J.: Current posttraumatic stress disorder and cardiovascular disease risk factors in Dutch Resistance veterans from World War II, *Psychotherapy Psychosomatics,* 1992; 57:164-171.

64. Litz, B., Fisher, L., Keane, T.: Physical health problems in post-traumatic stress disorder: A risk factor analysis. In Keane, T., Wolfe, J. (Co-Chairs), *Components of Health Risk in Veterans with Post-traumatic Stress Disorder.* Symposium presented at the annual American Psychological Association Meeting, San Francisco, CA, August, 1991.

65. Kaplan, J., Manuck, S., Williams, J., Strawn, W.: Psychosocial influences on atherosclerosis: Evidence for effects and mechanisms in nonhuman primates. In Blascovich, J., Katkin, E., Eds., *Cardiovascular reactivity to psychological stress and disease* (pp. 49-82), Washington, DC: American Psychological Association, 1993.

66. Wilson, S., van der Kolk, B., Burbridge, J., Fisler, R., Kradin, R.: Phenotype of blood lymphocytes in PTSD suggests chronic immune activation, *Psychosomatics,* 1999; 40:222-225.

67. Weiner, H.: *Psychobiology and Human Disease,* New York: Elisevier, 1977.

68. Weiner, H.: The dynamics of the organism: Implications of recent biological thought for psychosomatic theory and research, *Psychosomatic Medicine,* 1989; 51: 608-635.

69. Grotstein, J.: The psychology of powerlessness: Disorders of self-regulation and interactional regulation as a newer paradigm for psychopathology, *Psychoanalytic Inquiry,* 1986; 6:93-118.

70. Schore, A.: *Affect Regulation and the Origin of the Self: The Neurobiology of Emotional Development,* Hillsdale, NJ: Lawrence Erlbaum Associates, 1994, p. 440.

Chapter 7

1. Blanchard, E., Kolb, L., Prins, A., Gates, M., McCoy, G.: Changes in plasma norepinephrine to combat-related stimuli among Vietnam veterans with posttraumatic stress disorder, *Journal of Nervous and Mental Disease,* 1991; 179:6:371-373.

2. Beecher, H.: Pain in men wounded in battle, *Annals of Surgery,* 1946; 123: 96-105.

3. van der Kolk, B., Greenberg, M., Orr, S., Pitman, R.: Endogenous opioids and stress-induced analgesia in posttraumatic stress disorder, *Psychopharmocological Bulletin,*1989; 25:108-112.

4. Pattison, E., Kahan, J.: The deliberate self-harm syndrome, *American Journal of Psychiatry,*1983; 140:867-872.

5. Rosenthal, R., Rinzler, C., Wallsh, T., Klausner, E.: Wrist-cutting syndrome: The meaning of a gesture, *American Journal of Psychiatry,* 1972; 128:47-52.

6. Simpson, C., Porter, G.: Self-mutilation in children and adolescents, *Bulletin of the Meninger Clinic,* 1981; 45:428-438.

7. Russell, D.: *The Secret Trauma,* New York: Basic Books, 1986.

8. Silbert, M., Pines, A.: Sexual abuse as an antecedent to prostitution, *Child Abuse Neglect,* 1981; 5:407-411.

9. Schore, A.: *Affect Development and the Origin of the Self,* Hillsdale, NJ: Lawrence Erlbaum Associates, Inc., 1994.

10. Weiss, J., Glazer, H., Pohorecky, L., Brick, J., Miller N.: Effects of chronic exposure to stressors on subsequent avoidance-escape behavior and on brain norepinephrine, *Psychosomatic Medicine,* 1975; 37:522-524.

11. Cicchetti, D.: The emergence of developmental psychopathology, *Child Development,* 1984; 55:1-7.

12. Harlow, H., Zimmerman, R.: Affectional responses in infant monkeys, *Science,* 1959; 130:421-432.

13. Kling, A., Steklis, H.: A neural substrate for affiliative behavior in non-human primates, *Brain Behavioral Evolution,* 1976; 13:216-238.

14. Panksepp, J.: Toward a general psychobiological theory of emotions, *Behavioral Brain Science,*1982; 5:407-468.

15. Amir, S., Brown, Z., Amit, Z.: The role of endorphins in stress: Evidence and speculations, *Neuroscience Biobehavioral Review,* 1980; 4:77-86.

16. Solomon, R.: The opponent-process theory of acquired motivation: The costs of pleasure and the benefits of pain, *American Psychology,* 1980; 35:691-712.

17. Walker, L.: *The Battered Woman,* New York: Harper and Row, 1979.

18. Mitchell, D., Osborne, E., O'Boyle, M.: Habituation under stress: Shocked mice show nonassociative learning in a T-maze, *Behavioral Neural Biology,* 1985; 43:212-217.

19. Sheldon, A.: Preference for familiar vs. novel stimuli as a function of the familiarity of the environment, *Journal of Comparative Physiological Psychology,*1969; 67:517-521.

20. Erschak, G.: The escalation and maintenance of spouse abuse: A cybernetic model, *Victimology,* 1984; 9:247-253.

21. Carmen, E., Reiker, P., Mills, T.: Victims of violence and psychiatric illness, *American Journal of Psychiatry,* 1984; 141:378-379.

22. Jaffe, P., Wolfe, D., Wilson, S., Zak, L.: Family violence and child adjustment: A comparative analysis of girls' and boys' behavioral symptoms, *American Journal of Psychiatry,* 1986; 143:74-77.

23. Groth, A.: Sexual trauma in the life histories of sex offenders, *Victimology,* 1979; 4:6-10.

24. Seghorn, T., Boucher, R., Prentky, R.: Childhood sexual abuse in the lives of sexually aggressive offenders, *Journal of the American Academy of Child and Adolescent Psychiatry,* 1987; 26:262-267.

25. Perry, B., Pollard, R., Blakley, T., Baker, W., Vigilante, D.: Childhood trauma, the neurobiology of adaptation, and "use-dependent" development of the brain: How "states" become "traits," *Infant Mental Health Journal,* 1995; 16(4):271-291.

26. van der Kolk, B.: The compulsion to repeat the trauma: Re-enactment, revictimization, and masochism, *Psychiatric Clinics of North America,* 1989; 12(2):389-410.

Chapter 8

1. Janet, P.: *The Major Symptoms of Hysteria,* New York: Macmillan, 1920.

2. Freud, S., Breuer, J.: On the physical mechanism of hysterical phenomena. In Jones, E., Ed., *Sigmund Freud, MD, LLD. Collected Papers, Volume 1.* London: Hogarth Press, 1953, pp. 24-41.

3. Mayer-Gross, W.: On depersonalization, *British Journal of Medical Psychology,* 1935; 15:103-126.

4. Spiegal, D., Cardena, E.: Disintegrated experience: The dissociative disorders revisited, *Journal of Abnormal Psychology,* 1991; 100:366-378.

5. Bremner, J., Southwick, S., Brett, E., Fontana, A., Rosinheck, R., Charney, D.: Dissociation and posttraumatic stress disorder in Vietnam combat veterans, *American Journal of Psychiatry,* 1992; 149:328-332.

6. Putnam, F., Guroff, J., Silberman, E., Barban, L., Post, R.: The clinical phenomenology of multiple personality disorder: Review of 100 recent cases, *Journal of Clinical Psychiatry,* 1986; 47:285-293.

7. Christianson, S.: The relationship between induced arousal and amnesia, *Scandinavian Journal of Psychology,* 1984; 25:147-160.

8. Briere, J., Conte, J.: Self-reported amnesia for abuse in adults molested in childhood, *Journal of Traumatic Stress,* 1993; 6:21-31.

9. Pynoos, R., Frederick, C., Nader, K., Arroyo, W., Steinberg, A., Eth, S., Nunez, F., Fairbanks, L.: Life threat and posttraumatic stress disorder in school-age children, *Archives of General Psychiatry,* 1087; 44:1057-1063.

10. Terr, L.: Time sense following psychic trauma: A clinical study of ten adults and twenty children, *American Journal of Orthopsychiatry,* 1983; 53:244-261.

11. Mellman, T., Davis, G.: Combat-related flashbacks in posttraumatic stress disorder: Phenomenology and similarity to panic attacks, *Journal of Clinical Psychiatry,* 1985; 46:379-382.

12. van der Kolk, B.: The body keeps the score: Memory and the evolving psychobiology of posttraumatic stress, *Harvard Review of Psychiatry,* 1994; January/February:253-265.

13. Bremner, D., Scott, T., Delaney, R., Southwick, S., Mason, J., Johnson, D., Innis, J., McCarthy, G., Charney, D.: Deficits in short-term memory in posttraumatic stress disorder, *American Journal of Psychiatry,* 1993; 150(7):1015-1019.

14. Goldstein, G., van Kammen, W., Shelly, C., Miller, D., van Kammen, D.: Survivors of imprisonment in the Pacific theater during World War II, *American Journal of Psychiatry,* 1987; 144:1210-1213.

15. Sutker, P., Allain, A., Motsinger, P.: Minnesota Multiphasic Personality Inventory (MMPI)-derived psychopathology sub-types among former prisoners of

war (POWs): Replication and extension, *Journal of Psychopathology and Behavioral Assessment*, 1988; 10:129-140.

16. Thygesen, P., Hermann, I., Willanger, R.: Concentration camp survivors in Denmark: Persecution, disease, compensation, *Danish Medical Bulletin*, 1970; 17: 65-108.

17. Sutker, P., Winstead, D., Galina, Z., Allain, A.: Cognitive deficits and psychopathology among former prisoners of war and combat veterans of the Korean conflict, *American Journal of Psychiatry*, 1991; 148:67-72.

18. Bremner, J., Steinberg, M., Southwick, S., Johnson, D., Charney, D.: Use of the structured clinical interview for DSM-IV dissociative disorders for systematic assessment of dissociative symptoms in posttraumatic stress disorder, *American Journal of Psychiatry*, 1993; 150:1011-1014.

19. Zeitlin, S., McNally, R.: Implicit and explicit memory bias for threat in post-traumatic stress disorder, *Behaviour Research and Therapy*, 1991; 29:451-457.

20. Hilgard, E.: *Divided Consciousness: Multiple Controls in Human Thought and Action*, New York: Wiley, 1977.

21. Krystal, J., Bennett, A., Bremner, J., Southwick, S., Charney, D.: Toward a cognitive neuroscience of dissociation and altered memory functions in post-traumatic stress disorder. In Friedman, M.J., Charney, D.S., Deutch, A.Y., Eds., *Neurobiological and Clinical Consequences of Stress* (pp. 244-245), Philadelphia: Lippincott-Raven, 1995.

22. van der Kolk, B., van der Hart, O.: Pierre Janet and the breakdown of adaptation in psychological trauma, *American Journal of Psychiatry*, 1989; 146:1530-1540.

23. Bremner, J., Southwick, L., Brett, E., Fontana, A., Rosenheck, R., Charney, D.: Dissociation and posttraumatic stress disorder in Vietnam combat veterans, *American Journal of Psychiatry*, 1992; 149:328-332.

24. Holen, A.: The North Sea oil rig disaster. In Wilson, J., Raphael, B., Eds., *International Handbook of Traumatic Stress Syndromes* (pp. 471-479), New York: Plenum Press, 1993.

25. Cardena, E., Spiegel, D.: Dissociative reactions to the Bay Area earthquake, *American Journal of Psychiatry*, 1993; 150:474-478.

26. Kolb, L.: Neurophysiological hypothesis explaining posttraumatic stress disorder, *American Journal of Psychiatry*, 1987; 144:989-995.

27. McFarlane, A., Weber, D., Clark, C.: Abnormal stimulus processing in PTSD, *Biological Psychiatry*, 1993; 34:311-320.

28. Morgan, M., LeDoux, J.: Differential contributions of dorsal and ventral medial prefrontal cortex to the acquisition and extinction of conditioned fear in rats, *Behavioral Neuroscience*, 1995; 109:681-688.

29. Hamner, M., Loberbaum, J., George, M.: Potential role of the anterior cingulate cortex in PTSD: Review and hypothesis, *Depression and Anxiety*, 1999; 9:1-14.

30. van der Kolk, B.: The compulsion to repeat the trauma: Re-enactment, revictimization and masochism, *Psychiatric Clinics of North America*, 1989; 12:389-411.

31. American Psychiatric Association: *Diagnostic and Statistical Manual of Mental Disorders*, Fourth Edition (DSM-IV), Washington, DC: American Psychiatric Association, 1994.

32. Antelman, S., Caggiula, A., Kiss, D., Edwards, D., Kocan, D., Stiller, R.: Neurochemical and physiological effects of cocaine oscillate with sequential drug treatment: Possibly a major factor in drug variability, *Neuropsychopharmocology*, 1995; 12:297-306.

33. Caggiula, A., Antelman, S., Palmer, A., Kiss, S., Edwards, D. Kocan, D.: The effects of ethanol on striatal dopamine and frontal cortical D-[3H] aspartate efflux oscillate with repeated treatment: Relevance to individual differences in responsiveness, *Neuropsychopharmacology*, 1996; 15:125-132.

34. Antelman, S., Caggiula, A.: Oscillation follows drug implications, *Critical Review of Neurobiology*, 1996; 10:101-117.

35. Antelman, S., Caggiula, A., Gershon, S., Edwards. D., Austin, M., Kiss, S., Kocan, D.: Stressor-induced oscillation: A possible model of the bidirectional symptoms of PTSD, *New York Academy of Sciences*, 1997; 21:296-305.

36. Southwick, S., Yehuda, R., Wang, S.: Neuroendocrine alterations in posttraumatic stress disorder, *Psychiatric Annals*, 1998; 28:8:436-450.

37. Schore, A.: *Affect Regulation and the Origin of the Self*, Hillsdale, NJ: Lawrence Erlbaum Associates, 1994, pp. 204-209.

38. Porges, S.: Orienting in a defensive world: Mammalian modifcations of our evolutionary heritage. A polyvagal theory, *Psychophysiology*, 1995; 32:301-318.

39. Cannon, W.: "Voodoo" death, *Psychosomatic Medicine*, 1957; 19:182-190, reprinted from *American Anthropology*, 1942; 44:169.

40. Richter, C.: On the phenomenon of sudden death in animals and man, *Psychosomatic Medicine*, 1957; 19:191-198.

41. Hofer, M.: Cardiac respiratory function during sudden prolonged immobility in wild rodents, *Psychosomatic Medicine*, 1970; 32:633-647.

42. Koelman, J., Hilgevoord, A., Bour, L., Speelman, J., Ongerboer, B.: Soleus H-reflex tests in causalgia-dystonia compared with dystonia and mimicked dystonic posture, *Neurology*, 1999; 53:2196-2198.

43. Shuper, A., Zeharia, A., Mimouni, M.: Migraine headaches induced by sexual abuse, *Headache*, 1994; 34(4):237.

44. Gill, J., Stein, H.: More on sexual abuse and headaches, *Headache*, 1988; 28(2): 138.

45. Cwikel, J., Abdelyani, A., Goldsmith, J., Quastel, M., Yevelson, I.: Two-year follow up study of stress-related disorders among immigrants to Israel from the Chernobyl area, *Environmental Health Perspectives*, 1997; 105(6):1545-1550.

46. Perry, S., Tepperman, N., Greyson, D., Hilbert, L., Jimenez, J., Williams, J.: Reflex sympathetic dystrophy in hemiplegia, *Archives of Physical Medicine and Rehabilitation*, 1984; 65:442-446.

47. Dursun, E., Dursun, N., Ural, C., Cakci, A.: Glenohumeral joint subluxation and reflex sympathetic dystrophy in hemiplegic patients, *Archives of Physical Medicine and Rehabilitation*, 2000; 81:944-946.

Chapter 9

1. American Psychiatric Association: *Diagnostic and Statistical Manual of Mental Disorders,* Third Edition (DSM-III), Washington, DC: American Psychiatric Association, 1980.

2. American Psychiatric Association: *Diagnostic and Statistical Manual of Mental Disorders,* Third Edition, Revised (DSM-III-R), Washington, DC: American Psychiatric Association, 1987.

3. American Psychiatric Association: *Diagnostic and Statistical Manual of Mental Disorders,* Fourth Edition (DSM-IV), Washington, DC: American Psychiatric Association, 1994.

4. Helzer, J.E., Robins, L.N., McEvoy, L.: Post-traumatic stress disorder in the general population: Findings of the Epidemiologic Catchment Area survey, *New England Journal of Medicine,* 1987; 317(26):1630-1634.

5. Zohar, J., Sasson, Y., Amital, D., Iancu, J., Zinger, Y.: Current diagnostic and epidemiological insights in PTSD, *CNS Spectrums,* 1998; 3:7(2):12-14.

6. American Psychiatric Association: *Diagnostic and Statistical Manual of Mental Disorders,* First Edition (DSM-I), Washington, DC: American Psychiatric Association, 1952.

7. American Psychiatric Association: *Diagnostic and Statistical Manual of Mental Disorders,* Second Edition (DSM-II), Washington, DC: American Psychiatric Association, 1968.

8. Blanchard, E., Hickling, E.: *After the Crash,* Washington DC: American Psychological Association, 1997.

9. van der Kolk, B., Pelcovitz, D., Roth, S., Mandel, F., MacFarlane, A., Herman, J.: Dissociation, affect regulation and somatization: The complex nature of adaptation to trauma, *American Journal of Psychiatry,* 1996; 153(Supplement), 83-93.

10. Levine, P.: *Waking the Tiger,* Berkeley: North Atlantic Press, 1997, pp. 128-129.

11. Krystal, H.: Trauma and affect, *Psychoanalytic Study of the Child,* 1978; 33: 81-116.

12. Hobfoll, S.: *The Ecology of Stress,* New York: Hemisphere, 1988.

13. Breslau, N., Davis, G.: Post-traumatic stress disorder: The stressor criterion, *Journal of Nervous and Mental Disease,* 1987; 175:255-264.

14. Solomon, S., Canino, G.: The appropriateness of DSM-III-R criteria for post-traumatic stress disorder, *Comprehensive Psychiatry,* 1990; 31:227-237.

15. Norris, F.: Epidemiology of trauma: Frequency and impact of different potentially traumatic events on different demographic groups, *Journal of Consulting and Clinical Psychology,* 1992; 60(3):409-418.

16. Solomon, Z.: *Combat Stress Reaction: The Enduring Toll of War,* New York: Plenum Press, 1993.

17. Solomon, Z., Loar, N., McFarlane, A.: Acute posttraumatic reactions in soldiers and civilians. In van der Kolk, B., McFarlane, A., Weisaeth, L., Eds., *Traumatic Stress: The Effects of Overwhelming Experience on Mind, Body and Society,* New York: The Guilford Press, 1996, p. 104.

18. Kulka, R., Schlenger, W., Fairbank, H., Hough, R., Jordan, B., Marmar, C., Weiss, D.: *Trauma and the Vietnam War Generation*, New York: Brunner/Mazel, 1990.

19. Kessler, R., Sonnega, A., Bromet, E., Hughes, M., Nelson, C.: Posttraumatic stress disorder in the national comorbidity survey, *Archives of General Psychiatry*, 1995; 52:1048-1060.

20. Solomon, Z.: Somatic complaints, stress reaction and post-traumatic stress disorder: A 3-year follow-up study, *Behavioral Medicine*, 1988; 14:179-186.

21. Solomon, Z., Mikulincer, M., Kotler, M.: A two-year follow-up of somatic complaints among Isreali combat stress reaction casualties, 1987; 31:463-469.

22. Solomon, Z.: The psychological aftermath of combat stress reaction: An 18-year follow-up, Technical report, Israeli Ministry of Defense, 1994.

23. Kiser, K., Moll, J., Rankin, J.: Unexplained illness among Persian Gulf war veterans in an Air National Guard unit: Preliminary report, August, 1990–March, 1995, *Journal of the American Medical Association*, 1995; 274:16-17, and *Morbidity Mortality Weekly Report*, 1995; 44:443-447.

24. NIH Technology Assessment Workshop Panel. The Persian Gulf experience and health, *Journal of the American Medical Association*, 1994; 272:391-396.

25. Persian Gulf Veterans Coordinating Board. Unexplained illnesses among Desert Storm veterans, *Archives of Internal Medicine*, 1995; 155:262-268.

26. Amato, A., McVey, A., Cha, C., Matthews, E., Jackson, C., Kleingunther, R., Worley, L., Cornman, E., Kagan-Hallet, K.: Evaluation of neuromuscular symptoms in veterans of the Persian Gulf War, *Neurology*, 1997; 48:4-12

27. Bremner, J., Southwick, S., Johnson, D., Yehuda, R., Charney, D.: Childhood physical abuse and combat-related posttraumatic stress disorder in Vietnam veterans, *American Journal of Psychiatry*, 1993; 150(2):235-239.

28. Frye, J., Stockton, T:. Discriminant analysis of posttraumatic stress disorder among a group of Vietnam veterans: Analysis of premilitary, military and combat exposure influences, *American Journal of Psychiatry*, 1982; 139:52-56.

29. Solkoff, N., Gray, P., Keill, S.: Which Vietnam veterans develop posttraumatic stress disorder? *Journal of Clinical Psychology*, 1986; 42(5):687-698.

30. Keane, T., Scott, W., Chavoya, G., Lamparske, D., Fairbank, J.: Social support in Vietnam veterans with posttraumatic stress disorder: A comparative analysis, *Journal of Consulting and Clinical Psychology*, 1985; 53:95-102.

31. Foy, D., Sopprelle, R., Rueger, D., Carroll, E.: Etiology of posttraumatic stress disorder in Vietnam veterans: Analysis of premilitary, military and combat exposure influences, *Journal of Consulting and Clinical Psychology*, 1984; 52: 79-87.

32. Snow, B., Stellman, J., Stellman, S., Sommer, J.: Post-traumatic stress disorder among American Legionaires in relation to combat experience in Vietnam: Associated and contributing factors, *Environmental Research*, 1988; 47:175-192.

33. Schore, A. *Affect Regulation and the Origin of the Self*, Hillsdale, NJ: Lawrence Erlbaum and Associates, 1994.

34. Perry, B., Pollard, R., Blakeley, T., Baker, W., Vigilante, D.: Childhood trauma, the neurobiology of adaptation, and "use-dependent" development of the brain: How "states" become "traits," *Infant Mental Health Journal,* 1995; 16(4):271-291.

35. Grigsby, J., Hartlaub, G.: Procedural learning and the development and stability of character, *Perceptual and Motor Skills,* 1994; 79:355-370.

36. Seghorn, T., Boucher, R., Prentky, R.: Childhood sexual abuse in the lives of sexually aggressive offenders, *Journal of the American Academy of Child and Adolescent Psychiatry,* 1987; 26:262-267.

37. Lewis, D., Pincus, J., Bard, B, Richardson, E., Pricep, L., Feldman, M., Yeager, C.: Neuropsychiatric, psychoeducational and family characteristics of 14 juveniles condemned to death in the United States, *American Journal of Psychiatry,* 1988; 145:584-589.

38. Perry, B.: Evolution of symptoms following traumatic events in children (Abstract), *Proceedings of the 148th Annual Meeting of the American Psychiatric Association,* Miami, FL, 1995.

39. Ford, J., Kidd, P.: Early childhood trauma and disorders of extreme stress as predictors of treatment outcome with chronic posttraumatic stress disorder, *Journal of Traumatic Stress,* 1998; 11(4):743-761.

40. McFarlane, A., van der Kolk, B.: Trauma and its challenge to society. In van der Kolk, B., McFarlane, A., Weisaeth, L, Eds., *Traumatic Stress: The Effects of Overwhelming Experience on Mind, Body and Society* (pp. 36-39), New York: The Guilford Press, 1996.

41. Springs, F., Friedrich, W.: Health risk behaviors and medical sequelae of childhood sexual abuse, *Mayo Clinic Proceedings,* 1992; 67:527.

42. Tennant, C.: Life events and psychological morbidity: The evidence from prospective studies, *Psychological Medicine,* 1983; 13:483-486.

43. Wood, C.: Sexual abuse during childhood and adolescence and its effects on the physical and emotional quality of life of the survivor: A review of the literature, *Military Medicine,* 1996; 161:582-587.

44. National Victim Center: Crime and victimization in America: Statistical overview, Arlington, VA, 1993.

45. Resnick, H., Kilpatrick, D., Best, C., Kramer, T.: Vulnerability-stress factors in development of posttraumatic stress disorder, *Journal of Nervous and Mental Disease,* 1992: 180:424-430.

46. McFarlane, A.: The aetiology of post-traumatic morbidity: Predisposing, precipitating and perpetuating factors, *British Journal of Psychiatry,* 1989; 154:221-228.

47. Breslau, N., Andreski, P, Peterson, E.: Posttraumatic stress disorder in an urban population of young adults: Risk factors for chronicity, *American Journal of Psychiatry,* 1992; 149:671-675.

48. Carlson, E., Rosser-Hogan, R.: Trauma experiences, posttraumatic stress, dissociation and depression in Cambodian refugees, *American Journal of Psychiatry,* 1991; 148:1548-1551.

49. Ramsey, R., Gorst-Unsworth, C., Turner, S.: Psychiatric morbidity in survivors of organized state violence including torture: A retrospective series, *British Journal of Psychiatry*,1993; 162:55-59.

50. Kessler, R., Sonnega, A, Bromet, E., Hughes, M., Nelson, C.: Posttraumatic stress disorder in the national comorbidity survey, *Archives of General Psychiatry*, 1995; 51:1048-1060.

51. Resnick, H., Kilpatrick, D., Dansky, B., Saunders, B., Best, C.: Prevalence of civilian trauma and posttraumatic stress disorder in a representative national sample of women, *Journal of Consulting and Clinical Psychology*, 1993; 61:984-991.

52. Norris, F.: Screening for traumatic stress: A scale for use in the general population, *Journal of Applied Social Psychology*, 1990; 20:1704-1718.

53. International Federation of Red Cross and Red Crescent Societies: *World Disaster Report, 1993*. Dordrecht, The Netherlands: Martinus Nijhoff, 1993.

54. Breslau, N.: Epidemiology of trauma and posttraumatic stress disorder in psychological trauma. In Yehuda, R., Ed., *Psychological Trauma* (Review of Psychiatry, Vol. 17) (pp. 1-29), Washington, DC: American Psychiatric Association Press, 1998.

55. Koss, M., Burkhart, B.: A conceptual analysis of rape victimization, *Psychology of Women Quarterly*, 1989; 13:27-40.

56. Warshaw, R.: I Never Called It Rape: The Ms. Report on Recognizing, Fighting, and Surviving Date and Acquaintance Rape, New York: Harper and Row, 1998.

57. Koss, M., Dinero, T., Seibel, C.: Stranger and acquaintance rape: Are there differences in the victim's experience? *Psychology of Women Quarterly*, 1988; 12:1-24.

58. Bernstein, S., Small, S.: Psychodynamic factors in surgery, *Journal of Mount Sinai Hospital*, 1951; 17:938-958.

59. Deutsch, H.: Some psychoanalytic observations in surgery, *Psychosomatic Medicine*, 1942; 4:105-115.

60. Dumas, R.: Psychological preparation for surgery, *American Journal of Nursing*, 1963; 63:52-55.

61. Eckenoff, J.: Some preoperative warnings of operating room deaths, *New England Journal of Medicine*, 1956; 255:1075-1079.

62. Giller, D.: Some psychological factors in recovery from surgery, *Hospital Topics*, 1963; 41:83-85.

63. Williams, J., Jones, J.: Psychophysiological responses to anesthesia and operation, *Journal of the American Medical Association*, 1968; 203:415-417.

64. Williams, J., Jones, J., Williams, B.: A physiological measure of preoperative anxiety, *Psychosomatic Medicine*, 1969; 31:6:522-527.

65. Auerbach, S.: Trait-state anxiety and adjustment to surgery, *Journal of Consulting and Clinical Psychology*, 1973; 40:264-271.

66. Speilberger, S., Auerbach, S., Wadsworth, A., Dunn, T., Taulbee, E.: Emotional reactions to surgery, *Journal of Consulting and Clinical Psychology*, 1973; 40:33-38.

67. Martinez-Urrutia, A.: Anxiety and pain in surgical patients, *Journal of Consulting and Clinical Psychology*, 1975; 43:437-442.

68. Moote, S., Skinner, M., Grace, D., Knill, R.: Profound disruption of sleep in the first week after abdominal surgery, *Canadian Anaesthetists' Society Journal,* 1986; 33:S105.

69. Knill, R., Moote, C., Skinner, M., Rose, E.: Anesthesia with abdominal surgery leads to intense REM sleep during the first postoperative week, *Anesthesiology,* 1990; 73:52-61.

70. Brimacombe, J., Macfie, M., Peri-operative nightmares in surgical patients, *Anesthesia,* 1993; 48:527-529.

71. Kutz, I., Garb, R., David, D.: Post-traumatic stress disorder following myocardial infarction, *General Hospital Psychiatry,* 1998; 10:169-176.

72. Doerfler, L., Pbert, L., DeCosimo, D.: Symptoms of posttraumatic stress disorder following myocardial infarction and coronary artery bypass surgery, *General Hospital Psychiatry,* 1994; 16:193-194.

73. Schreiber, S., Galai-Gat, T.: Uncontrolled pain following physical injury as the core-trauma in post-traumatic stress disorder, *Pain,* 1993; 54:107-110.

74. Alter, C., Pelcovitz, D., Axelrod, A., Goldenberg, B., Harris, H., Meyers, B., Grofois, B., Mandel, F., Septimus, A., Kaplan, S.: Identification of PTSD in cancer survivors, *Psychosomatics,* 1996; 37:137-143.

75. Cella, D., Mahon, S., Donovan, M.: Cancer recurrence as a traumatic event, *Behavioral Medicine,* 1990; 16:15-22.

76. Cordova, M., Andryskowsky, M., Kenady, D., McGrath, P., Sloan, D., Redd, W.: Frequency and correlates of posttraumatic-stress-disorder-like symptoms after treatment for breast cancer, *Journal of Consulting Clinical Psychology,* 1995; 63:981-986.

77. Kelly, B., Raphael, B., Smithers, M., Swanson, C., Reid, C., McLeod, R., Thomson, D., Walpole, E.: Psychological responses to malignant melanoma: An investigation of traumatic stress reactions to life-threatening illness, *General Hospital Psychiatry,* 1995; 17:126-136.

78. Tjemsland, L., Soreide, J., Malt, U.: Traumatic distress symptoms in early breast cancer I: Acute response to diagnosis, *Psycho-Oncology,* 1996; 5:1-8.

79. Tjemsland, L., Soreide, J., Malt, U.: Traumatic distress symptoms in early breast cancer II: Outcome six weeks post surgery, *Psycho-Oncology,* 1996; 5:295-303.

80. Tjemsland, L., Soreide, J., Malt, U.: Traumatic distress symptoms in early breast cancer III: Breast cancer research and treatment, *Psycho-Oncology,* 1998; 47: 141-151.

81. Dossey, L.: *Meaning and Medicine: Lessons from a Doctor's Tales of Breakthrough and Healing,* New York: Bantam Books, 1991.

82. Siegel, B.: *Love, Medicine and Miracles,* New York: Harper & Row, 1986.

83. van der Kolk, B., Perry, J., Herman, J.: Childhood origins of destructive behavior, *American Journal of Psychiatry,* 1991; 148:1665-1671.

84. Blacher, R.: On awakening during surgery: A syndrome of traumatic neurosis, *Journal of the American Medical Association,* 1975; 234:67-68.

85. Meyer, B., Blacher, R.: A traumatic neurotic reaction induced by succinylcholine chloride, *New York State Journal of Medicine,* 1961; 61:1255-1261.

86. Cheek, D.: Surgical memory and reaction to careless conversation, *American Journal of Clinical Hypnosis,* 1964; 6:237-240.

87. Osterman, J., van der Kolk, B.: Awareness during anesthesia and posttraumatic stress disorder, *General Hospital Psychiatry,* 1998; 20:274-281.

88. Schwendler, D., Kunze-Kronawitter, P., Dietrich, S., Klasing, H., Madler, C.: Conscious awareness during general anaesthesia: Patient's perceptions, emotions, cognition and reactions, *British Journal of Anaesthesia,* 1998; 80:133-139.

89. Moerman, N., Bonke, B., Oosting, J.: Awareness and recall during general anesthesia: Facts and feelings, *Anesthesiology,* 1993; 79:454-464.

90. Heneghan, C.: Clinical and medicolegal aspects of conscious awareness during anesthesia, *International Anesthesiology Clinics,* 1993; 31:1-11.

91. van der Kolk, B., Fisler, R.: Dissociation and the fragmentary nature of traumatic memories: Overview and exploratory study, *Journal of Traumatic Stress,* 1995; 8:505-525.

92. Pernick, M.: *A Calculus of Suffering: Pain, Professionalism, and Anesthesia in the 9th Century,* New York: Columbia University Press, 1985.

93. Chamberlain, D.: Birth and the origins of violence, *Journal of Pre- and Perinatal Psychology,* 1995; 10(2):57-74.

94. Leader, L., Baillie, P., Martin, B., Vermeulen, E.: The assessment and significance of habituation to a repeated stimulus by the human fetus, *Early Human Development,* 1982; 18:307-319.

95. Rovee-Collier, C., Lipsitt, L.: Learning, adaptation and memory in the newborn. In Stratton, P., Ed., Psychobiology of the human newborn, London:Wiley & Sons, 1982, pp. 147-190.

96. Iannirubito, A., Tajani, E.: Ultrasonographic study of fetal movements, *Seminars in Perinatology,* 1981; 5(2):175-181.

97. Giannakoulopoulos, X., Sepulveda, W., Kourtis, P., Glover, V., Fisk, N.: Fetal plasma cortisol and B-endorphin response to intrauterine needling, *Lancet,* 1994; 344:77-81.

98. DeCasper, A., Lecanuet, J., Busnel, M., Granier-Deferre, C., Mangeais, R.: Fetal reactions to recurrent maternal speech, *Infant Behavior and Development,* 1994; 17(2):159-164.

99. DeCasper, A., Lecanuet, J-P., Busnel, M-C., Granier-Deferre, C., Mangeais, R., Fetal reactions to recurrent maternal speech, *Infant Behavior and Development,* 1994; 17(2):159-164.

100. Raine, A., Brennan, P., Mednick, S.: Birth complications combined with early maternal rejection at age one year predispose to violent crime at age 18, *Archives of General Psychiatry,* 1994; 51:948-988.

101. Taddio, A., Goldblach, M., Ipp, M., Stevens, B., Koren, G.: Effect of neonatal circumcision on pain responses during vaccination of boys, *Lancet,* 1995; 345: 291-292.

102. American Academy of Pediatrics: Circumsion policy statement, *Pediatrics,* 1999; 103(3):686-693.

103. Anand, K., Phil, D., Ward-Platt, M.: Neonatal and pediatric stress responses to anesthesia and operation, *International Anesthesiology Clinics*, 1988; 26(3):218-225.

104. Jackson, K., Winkley, A., Faust, O., Cermak, E., Burtt, M.: Behavior changes indicating emotional trauma in tonsillectomized children, *Journal of the American Medical Association*, 1952; 149:1536.

Chapter 10

1. American Psychiatric Association: *Diagnostic and Statistical Manual of Mental Disorders*, Third Edition (DSM-III), Washington, DC: American Psychiatric Association, 1980.

2. Grinker, R., Speigel, J. *Men Under Stress*, Phildelphia: Blakiston, 1945.

3. Fischer, H., Wik.,G., Fredrikson, M.: Functional neuroanatomy of robbery reexperience: Affective memories studied with PET, *Neuroreport*, 1996; 7(13): 2081-2086.

4. van der Kolk, B., McFarlane, A., van der Hart, O.: A general approach to treatment of posttraumatic stress disorder. In van der Kolk, B., McFarlane, A., Weisaeth, L., Eds., *Traumatic Stress: The Effects of Overwhelming Experience on Mind, Body and Society* (pp. 417-440), New York: The Guilford Press, 1996.

5. van der Hart, O., Steele, K., Brown, P.: The treatment of traumatic memories: Synthesis, realization and integration, *Dissociation*, 1993; 6:162-180.

6. Cooper, N., Chum, G.: Imaginal flooding as a supplementary treatment for PTSD in combat veterans: A controlled study, *Behavioral Therapy*, 1989; 20(3):381-391.

7. Resick, P., Schnicke, M.: Cognitive processing therapy for sexual assault victims, *Journal of Consulting and Clinical Psychology*, 1992; 60(5):748-756.

8. Brom, D., Kleber, R.: Prevention of post-traumatic stress disorders, *Journal of Traumatic Stress*, 1989; 2(3):335-351.

9. Foa, E., Rothbaum, B., Molnar, C.: Cognitive-behavioral treatment of posttraumatic stress disorder. In Friedman, M., Charney, D., Deutch, A., Eds., *Neurobiological and Clinical Consequences of Stress: From Normal Adaptation to Posttraumatic Stress Disorder* (pp. 483-491), New York: Raven Press, 1995.

10. Pitman, R., Altman, B., Greenwald E., Longpre, R., Macklin, M., Poire, R., Steketee, G.: Psychiatric complications during flooding therapy for posttraumatic stress disorder, *Journal of Clinical Psychiatry*, 1991; 52:17-20.

11. Foa, E., Davidson, J., Rothbaum, B.: Treatment of posttraumatic stress disorder. In Gabbard, O., Ed., *Treatment of Psychiatric Disorders: The DSM-IV Edition*, (pp. 1499-1519). Washington DC: American Psychiatric Press, 1995.

12. Rothbaum, B., Foa, E.: Cognitive-behavioral techniques for posttraumatic stress disorder. In van der Kolk, B., McFarlane, A., Weisaeth, L., Eds., *Traumatic Stress: The Effects of Overwhelming Experience on Mind, Body and Society* (pp. 491-509), New York: The Guilford Press, 1996.

13. Rothbaum, B., Foa, E.: Exposure therapy for PTSD, *PTSD Research Quarterly* (p. 3), The National Center for Post-Traumatic Stress Disorder, White River Junction, VT, Spring 1999.

14. Shapiro, F.: Efficacy of the Eye Movement Desensitization procedure in the treatment of traumatic memories, *Journal of Traumatic Stress,* 1989; 2:199-223.

15. Wilson, S., Becker, L., Tinker, R.: Eye movement desensitization and reprocessing (EMDR) treatment for psychologically traumatized individuals, *Journal of Consulting and Clinical Psychology,* 1995; 63(6):928-937.

16. Wilson, S., Becker, L., Tinker, T.: Fifteen-month follow-up of eye movement desensitization and reprocessing (EMDR) treatment for posttraumatic stress disorder and psychological trauma, *Journal of Consulting and Clinical Psychology,* 1997; 65(6):1047-1056.

17. Rothbaum, B.: A controlled study of eye movement desensitization and reprocessing in the treatment of posttraumatic stress disordered sexual assault victims, *Bulletin of the Menninger Clinic,* 1997; 61:317-334.

18. Jensen, J.: An investigation of eye movement desensitization and reprocessing (EMDR) as a treatment for posttraumatic stress disorder (PTSD) symptoms of Vietnam combat veterans, *Behavioral Therapy,* 1994; 25:311-325.

19. Carlson, J., Chemtob, C., Rusnak, K., Hedlund, N., Muraoka, M.: Eye movement desensitization and reprocessing (EMDR) treatment for combat-related posttraumatic stress disorder, *Journal of Traumatic Stress,* 1998; 11:3-24.

20. Vaughn, K., Armstrong, M., Gold, R., O'Connor, N., Jenneke, W., Tarrier, N.: A trial of eye movement desensitization compared to image habituation training and applied muscle relaxation in post-traumatic stress disorder, *Journal of Behavior Therapy and Experimental Psychiatry,* 1994; 25:283-291.

21. Devilly, G., Spence, S.: The relative efficacy and treatment distress of EMDR and a cognitive behavioral trauma treatment protocol in the amelioration of posttraumatic stress disorder, *Journal of Anxiety Disorders,* 1999; 13:131-157.

22. Cusack, K., Spates, C.: The cognitive dismantling of eye movement desensitization and reprocessing (EMDR) treatment of posttraumatic stress disorder PTSD, *Journal of Anxiety Disorders,* 1999; 13:87-89.

23. Wilson, D., Silver, S., Cove, W., Foster, S.: Eye movement desensitization and reprocessing: Effectiveness and autonomic correlates, *Journal of Behavioral Therapy and Experimental Psychiatry,* 1996; 27:219-229.

24. Pitman, R., Orr, S., Altman, B., Longpre, R., Poire, R., Macklin, M.: Emotional processing during eye movement desensitization and reprocessing therapy of Vietnam veterans with chronic posttraumatic stress disorder, *Comprehensive Psychiatry,* 1996; 37:419-429.

25. Shapiro, F.: *Eye Movement Desensitization and Reprocessing: Basic Principles, Protocols and Procedures,* New York: The Guilford Press, 1995.

26. Nicosia, G.: A mechanism for dissociation suggested by the quantitative analysis of electroencephalography. Paper presented at the International EMDR Annual Conference, Sunnyvale, CA, March, 1994.

27. van der Kolk, B.: Personal communication.

28. Bergmann, U.: Speculations on the neurobiology of EMDR, *Traumatology,* 1998; 4:1, Article 2.

29. Levine, P.: *Waking the Tiger,* 1997, Berkeley, CA: North Atlantic Press.

30. Cameron-Bandler, L.: *They Lived Happily Ever After,* Cupertino, CA: Meta Publications, 1978.

31. Callahan, R.: *The Five Minute Phobia Cure,* Wilmington, DE: Enterprise, 1985.

32. Gerbode, F.: Presentation during conference on "Active Ingredients in Efficient Treatments of PTSD," Florida State University, Tallahassee, FL, May 12, 1995.

33. Rosenthal, D., Frank, J.: Psychotherapy and the placebo effect, *Psychological Bulletin,* 1956; 53(4):294-302.

34. Goleman, D.: *Vital Lies, Simple Truths: The Psychology of Self-Deception,* New York: Simon & Schuster, 1985.

35. Cannon, W.: Voodoo death, *American Anthropologist,* 1942; 4:169-181.

36. Kardiner, A.: *The Traumatic Neurosis of War,* New York: Hoeber, 1941.

37. Guidotti, A., Baraldi, M., Leon, A., Costa., E.: Benzodiazepines: A tool to study the biochemical and neurophysiological basis of anxiety, *Federal Proceedings,*1980; 39:1039-1042.

38. Tietz, E., Gomaz, F., Berman, R.: Amygdala kindled seizure stage is related to altered benzodiazepine binding site density, *Life Science,* 1985; 36:183-190.

39. Risse, S., Whitters., A., Burke, J., Chen, S., Scurfield, R., Raskind, M.: Severe withdrawal symptoms after discontinuation of alprazolam in eight patients with combat-induced post-traumatic stress disorder, *Journal of Clinical Psychiatry,* 1990; 51(15):206-209.

40. Feldman, T.: Alprazolam in the treatment of post-traumatic stress disorder [letter], *Journal of Clinical Psychiatry,* 1987; 48:216-217.

41. Lowenstein, R., Hornstein, N, Farber, B.: Open trial of clonazepam in the treatment of post-traumatic stress disorder, *Dissociation,* 1988; 1:3-12.

42. Wells, G., Chu, C., Johnson, T., Nasdahl, C., Ayubi, M., Sewell, E., Statham, P.: Buspirone in the treatment of post-traumatic stress disorder, *Pharmacotherapy,* 1991; 11(4):340-343.

43. Davidson, J., Kudler, H., Smith, R., Mahoney, L., Lipper, S., Gammett, E., Saunders, W., Cavenar, J.: Treatment of post-traumatic stress disorder with amitriptyline and placebo, *Archives of General Psychiatry,* 1990; 47:259-266.

44. Davidson, J., Kudler, H., Saunders, W., Erickson, L., Smith, R., Stein, R., Lipper, S., Hammett, E., Mahoney, L., Cavenar., J.: Predicting response to amitriptyline in posttraumatic stress disorder, *American Journal of Psychiatry,* 1992; 150(7): 1024-1029.

45. Frank, J., Kosten, T., Giller, E., Dan, E.: A randomized clinical trial of phenelzine and imipramine for post-traumatic stress disorder, *American Journal of Psychiatry,* 1988; 145:128-129.

46. Kosten, T., Frank, J., Dan, E., McDougle, C., Giller, E.: Phamacotherapy for posttraumatic stress disorder using phenelzine or imipramine, *Journal of Nervous and Mental Disease,* 1991; 177(6):366-370.

47. Reist, C., Kauffmann, C., Haier, R., Sangdahl, C., Demet, E., Chicz-Demet, A., Nelson, J.: A controlled trial of desipramine in 18 men with post-traumatic stress disorder, *American Journal of Psychiatry,* 1989; 146:513-516.

48. Lipper, S., Davidson, J., Grady, T., Edingar, J., Hammett, E., Mahoney, S., Cavenar, J.: Preliminary study of carbamazepine in post-traumatic stress disorder, *Psychosomatics*, 1986; 27:849-854.

49. Fesler, F.: Valproate in combat-related post-traumatic stress disorder, *Journal of Clinical Psychiatry*, 1991; 52(9):361-364.

50. Kolb, L., Burris, B., Griffiths, S.: Propranolol and clonidine in the treatment of chronic posttraumatic stress of war. In van der Kolk, B., Ed., *Posttraumatic Stress Disorder: Psychological and Biolological Sequelae* (pp.97-107), Washington, DC: American Psychiatry Press, 1984.

51. Famularo, R., Kinscherff, R., Fenton, T.: Propranolol treatment for childhood posttraumatic stress disorder, acute type, *American Journal of Diseases of Children*, 1988; 142:1244-1247.

52. Perry, B.: Neurobiological sequelae of childhood trauma: PTSD in children. In Murburg, M., Ed., *Catecholamine Function in Post-traumatic Stress Disorder: Emerging Concepts* (pp. 233-255), Washington, DC: American Psychiatric Press, 1994.

53. Kinzie, J.: Therapeutic approaches to traumatized Cambodian refugees, *Journal of Traumatic Stress*, 1989; 2:75-91.

54. van der Kolk, B., Dryfuss, D., Michaels, M., Berkowitz, R., Saxe, G., Goldenberg, I.: Fluoxitine in post-traumatic stress disorder, *Journal of Clinical Psychiatry*, 1994; 55:517-522.

55. Friedman, M.: A guide to the literature on pharmacotherapy for PTSD, *PTSD Research Quarterly*, Winter 2000; 11(1):1-7.

56. Pitman, R., van der Kolk, B., Orr, S., Greenberg, M.: Naloxone-reversible analgesic response to combat-related stimuli in post-traumatic stress disorder, *Archives of General Psychiatry*, 1990; 47:541-544.

57. Glover, H.: Emotional numbing: A possible endorphin-mediated phenomenon associated with post-traumatic stress disorder and other allied psychopathologic states, *Journal of Traumatic Stress*, 1992; 5:643-675.

58. Glover, H.: A preliminary trial of nalmefene for the treatment of emotional numbing in combat veterans with post-traumatic stress disorder, *Israeli Journal of Psychiatry Related Sciences*, 1993; 30(4):255-263.

59. Billis, L., Kreisler, K.: Treatment of flashbacks with naltrexone, *American Journal of Psychiatry*, 1993; 150(9):1430.

60. van der Kolk, B., van der Hart, O., Burbridge, J.: Approaches to the treatment of PTSD. In Hobfall, S., De Vries, W. Eds., *Extreme Stress and Communities; Impact and Intervention* (pp. 421-443). NATO Asi Series, Series D, Behavioral and Social Sciences, Volume 80, 1995.

Chapter 11

1. Bell, I., Miller, C., Schwartz, G.: An olfactory-limbic model of multiple chemical sensitivity syndrome: Possible relationships to kindling and affective spectrum disorders, *Biological Psychiatry*, 1992; 32:218-242.

2. Miller, L.: Neurosensitization: A pathophysiological model for traumatization disability syndromes, *The Journal of Cognitive Rehabilitation,* 1997; November/December:12-23.

3. Pace, J., Nagle, D.: Piriform syndrome, *Western Journal of Medicine,* 1976; 124: 435-439.

4. van der Kolk, B: The body keeps the score: Approaches to the psychobiology of posttraumatic stress disorder. In van der Kolk, B., McFarlane, A., Weisaeth, L. Eds., *Traumatic Stress,* New York: The Guilford Press, 1996, p. 293.

5. Rauch, S., van der Kolk, B., Fisler, R., Alpert, N., Orr., S., Savage. C., Fischman, A., Jenike, M., Pitman, R.: A symptom provocation study of posttraumatic stress disorder using positron emission tomography and script-driven imagery, *Archives of General Psychiatry,* 1996; 53:380-387.

6. Cleveland, S.E.: Personality dynamics in torticollis, *Journal of Nervous and Mental Disease,* 1961; 129:150-161.

7. Tibbets, R.W.: Spasmodic torticollis, *Journal of Nervous and Mental Disease,* 1971; 15:461-469.

8. Matthews, W.B., Beasley, P., Parry-Jones, W., Garland, G.: Spasmodic torticollis: A combined clinical study, *Journal of Neurology, Neurosurgery and Psychiatry,* 1978; 41:485-492.

9. Porges, S.: Orienting in a defensive world: Mammalian modifications of our evolutionary heritage. A polyvagal theory, *Psychophysiology,* 1995; 32:301-308.

Index

Page numbers followed by the letter "f" indicate figures.

Order Your Own Copy of
This Important Book for Your Personal Library!

THE BODY BEARS THE BURDEN
Trauma, Dissociation, and Disease

_____in hardbound at $59.95 (ISBN: 0-7890-1245-6)

_____in softbound at $39.95 (ISBN: 0-7890-1246-4)

COST OF BOOKS_____

OUTSIDE USA/CANADA/
MEXICO: ADD 20%____

POSTAGE & HANDLING_____
(US: $4.00 for first book & $1.50
for each additional book)
Outside US: $5.00 for first book
& $2.00 for each additional book)

SUBTOTAL_____

in Canada: add 7% GST____

STATE TAX____
(NY, OH & MIN residents, please
add appropriate local sales tax)

FINAL TOTAL____
(If paying in Canadian funds,
convert using the current
exchange rate, UNESCO
coupons welcome.)

❑ **BILL ME LATER:** ($5 service charge will be added)
(Bill-me option is good on US/Canada/Mexico orders only;
not good to jobbers, wholesalers, or subscription agencies.)

❑ Check here if billing address is different from
shipping address and attach purchase order and
billing address information.

Signature_____

❑ **PAYMENT ENCLOSED:** $_____

❑ **PLEASE CHARGE TO MY CREDIT CARD.**

❑ Visa ❑ MasterCard ❑ AmEx ❑ Discover
❑ Diner's Club ❑ Eurocard ❑ JCB

Account # _____

Exp. Date_____

Signature_____

Prices in US dollars and subject to change without notice.

NAME_____

INSTITUTION_____

ADDRESS_____

CITY_____

STATE/ZIP_____

COUNTRY_____ COUNTY (NY residents only)_____

TEL_____ FAX_____

E-MAIL_____

May we use your e-mail address for confirmations and other types of information? ❑ Yes ❑ No
We appreciate receiving your e-mail address and fax number. Haworth would like to e-mail or fax special
discount offers to you, as a preferred customer. **We will never share, rent, or exchange your e-mail address
or fax number.** We regard such actions as an invasion of your privacy.

Order From Your Local Bookstore or Directly From
The Haworth Press, Inc.
10 Alice Street, Binghamton, New York 13904-1580 • USA
TELEPHONE: 1-800-HAWORTH (1-800-429-6784) / Outside US/Canada: (607) 722-5857
FAX: 1-800-895-0582 / Outside US/Canada: (607) 722-6362
E-mail: getinfo@haworthpressinc.com
PLEASE PHOTOCOPY THIS FORM FOR YOUR PERSONAL USE.
www.HaworthPress.com

BOF00